D0886569

VIGILANCE

Vigilance

An Anesthesiologist's Notes on
Thriving in Uncertainty

Nabil Othman, MD

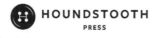

HOUNDSTOOTH
PRESS

VIGILANCE
An Anesthesiologist's Notes on Thriving in Uncertainty

ISBN   978-1-5445-2106-0 *Hardcover*
        978-1-5445-2105-3 *Paperback*
        978-1-5445-2104-6 *Ebook*

For my mother, Patricia McLeish.

All the good things in me are because of you.

Table of Contents

"*Though much is taken, much abides; and though
We are not now that strength which in old days
Moved earth and heaven; that which we are, we are;
One equal temper of heroic hearts,
Made weak by time and fate, but strong in will
To strive, to seek, to find, and not to yield.*"

—*Ulysses* by Alfred, Lord Tennyson (1842)

Introduction

Between my first and second years of medical school, I had three months off to do whatever I wanted. Some students completed clinical externships, some backpacked in Europe, and I chose to study blood clotting in pediatric cardiac surgery patients. In addition to my laboratory research, I rounded with the critical care team in the pediatric intensive care unit (PICU). It was there I met someone I will never forget.

A five-year-old boy named John had been admitted the previous night after nearly drowning in a bathtub. When I first saw him, he was lying on his back with his eyes closed. His hospital gown had elephants on it. I felt like I was peeking into the bedroom of a sleeping child. By the bedside, his mother held his hand and sobbed silently.

As I looked around the PICU, I noticed other rooms similar to John's: 24 glass boxes neatly arranged in a U-shape around a common computer workspace. Doctors were recording and interpreting patient data, looking for patterns of improvement or deterioration. The various monitor tones, ventilator breaths, computer keystrokes, and quiet conversations merged into an emotionless symphony.

When it was time for rounds, I was surprised by the topics of discussion. Our team focused on hypothetical catastrophes instead of what was actually happening to their patients. I noticed ICU physicians—who are supposed to be the best-trained doctors in the hospital—seemed obsessed with what they didn't know. They talked about arterial blood gases and acute respiratory distress syndrome as they played with the ventilator like a new video game. I spent my nights in the library learning how to interpret the endless data, wondering why we were collecting all these seemingly useless numbers.

Over the course of three days, John's lungs improved, and his breathing tube was removed. Still, the ICU physicians obsessed over dangerous, uncommon events that never happened. Couldn't they see John was improving? Their vigilance seemed out of proportion to the situation.

On my fifth day at the hospital, our team gathered in front of John's room for our morning rounds. Just as I did on my first day, I peeked into his room. But this time, he woke up, rose to his feet, and walked energetically back and forth in his crib! When he came to the side of the crib facing the doorway, he looked at me with the silly, innocent smile of a happy, well-adjusted five-year old.

Suddenly, in the midst of the countless vital signs and machinery that often makes hospitals seem so grim, my eyebrows unfurled, my shoulders relaxed, and my pursed lips transformed so much that the corners of my eyes wrinkled. On two sides of the glass, John and I began to laugh together. It was a joyous moment, and years later in residency, I finally understood why the ICU physicians' management of uncertainty was the key to making it a reality.

§ ANESTHESIOLOGY, SYNERGY, AND BLACK SWANS §

During my third year of medical school, I decided to become an anesthesiologist. Anesthesiologists and intensivists have more than a few things in common: both manage vital functions when patients cannot do so themselves, both interpret complex physiologic changes in real time, and both prevent catastrophic events in uncertain situations. In fact, the ICU was invented by an anesthesiologist in 1952 when Danish anesthesiologist Dr. Bjørn Ibsen applied operating room ventilation strategies to a ward of paralyzed polio patients in Copenhagen, Denmark.[1]

Several features make anesthesiology unique from other medical specialties. Our patient is always minutes away from death, and we must tolerate long periods of uncertainty interrupted by short bursts of unexpected intensity. We don't have time to consult anyone when complications occur. Working at a high speed with limited information, anesthesiologists learned how to think statistically about life-threatening conditions, such as bradycardia (low heart rate), hypoxia (not enough oxygen in the blood), and hypotension (low blood pressure). Over the years, we've become experts in the recognition, management, and prevention of emergencies occurring in high-uncertainty situations.

To save the lives of our patients, we've traded a simple cause-and-effect view of reality for a systems-based approach. Because we manage every organ system in the body—in real time, as they adapt to their internal changes and the changing surgical environment—we view the operating room in terms of synergy.

---

[1]   A summary can be found in the article "The Doctor Who Had to Innovate or Else" by Conor Friedersdorf, published in *The Atlantic*. A more academic version is "The Physiologic Challenges of the 1952 Copenhagen Poliomyelitis Epidemic and a Renaissance in Clinical Respiratory Physiology" by Dr. John West published in *The Journal of Applied Physiology*.

Synergy is the random, unintentional, and oftentimes invisible interactions between components of a system. As the number of components increases, synergistic interactions also increase. If the number of random interactions is high enough, they organize into events. A few events will cause desirable changes, most will cause no changes, and some will cause undesirable changes. Eventually, if enough synergy is present, a catastrophic event will destroy the system. In anesthesiology, the system is our patient, and the events are hypoxia, hypotension, and bradycardia. Outside of the operating room, these events are called Black Swans.

Black Swans are unpredictable, cataclysmic events retrospectively "obvious" due to psychological biases.[2] They are named after the ancient metaphor *rara avis*, which means "rare bird" in Latin. The metaphor was originally used as a compliment, meaning "one of a kind." In Ancient Greece, the expression evolved into Black Swan because, at that time, all known swans were white. Black Swan meant "someone so exceptional they have never been seen before."[3]

The modern expression—popularized by Nassim Taleb in 2007— means "a cataclysmic, unexpected, unpredictable event beyond the scope of human knowledge when it occurred." Black Swans are unexpected and unpredictable because they form from a random combination of synergistic interactions. Historical examples include the US stock market crash of 1929, World War II,

---

2   I highly recommend Nassim Taleb's *Incerto*, a series of four books about luck, uncertainty, probability, opacity, human error, risk, disorder, and decision making. My definition of a Black Swan is based on Part I of the second book in the series, *The Black Swan: The Impact of the Highly Improbable*.

3   I found a summary of Black Swan etymology at en.antiquitatem.com created by Antonio Marco Martinez, a retired professor of Latin. The specific page is titled "The White Blackbird and the Black Swan Are a Rare Avis (Rara Avis)."

and the sinking of the *Titanic*. Modern examples include the 9/11 New York City terrorist attack, the Sandy Hook Elementary School shooting, and COVID-19.

Over the last 70 years, the world's political and economic systems have become increasingly synergistic. In their complexity, these systems generate unprecedented wealth and innovation. However, that same complexity also makes them vulnerable to Black Swans. As we move forward, Black Swans will become more intense and occur more often because complexity and connectivity create more synergy, and more synergy creates Black Swans. Our world is a car accelerating toward the edge of a cliff.

So what does all this talk about synergy and Black Swans have to do with anesthesiology? Well, anesthesiologists already have a solution.

§ WHAT TO EXPECT IN THIS BOOK §

This book describes how anesthesiologists perceive the world, how they measure synergy to manage Black Swans, and how they ultimately prevent patient death. Our success speaks for itself. Anesthesia-related deaths in the United States—primarily from Black Swan events—have decreased from 640 per million anesthetics between 1948 and 1952 to 8.2 per million anesthetics between 1999 and 2005. A more recent study from 2018 showed an additional drop to 5.1 deaths per million anesthetics. This represents a 99.7% absolute reduction over 70 years.[4]

---

4   Anesthesia mortality varies slightly depending on the study. All of them show a steep drop from 1950 to 2020. The 1999–2005 study is "Is Anesthesia Dangerous?" by Dr. Andre Gottschalk. The 2018 study is "Perianesthetic and Anesthesia-Related Mortality in a Southeastern United States Population: A Longitudinal Review of a Prospectively Collected Quality Assurance Data Base" by Dr. Richard Pollard.

For perspective that means, on average, one patient dies because of anesthesia every 196,078 cases. Today, if I did three cases per day every day without taking any days off (1,095 cases/year), I would encounter a single death in 179 years. In the 1940s, I would encounter a death every 1.5 years. What's more, patients became exponentially more complex over the last 70 years: as physicians learned to treat disease, patients often developed additional more advanced diseases later in life that required more complicated treatment. Despite this positive feedback loop between patient treatment and increasing complexity, anesthesia has become exponentially safer.

The book is divided into four parts:

- Part I reveals how anesthesiologists recognize uncertainty: our philosophy of perception, our thinking patterns, and how we stay calm in dangerous situations. You will see what actually happens in the operating room, receive a firsthand account of my medical school training, and discover how cognitive psychology saves lives during emergencies.
- Part II depicts how anesthesiologists manage Black Swans: our early recognition of problems, how we extend the time horizon of catastrophic events, and how we protect essential systems of the body. You will see the seconds between life and death, learn about the history of anesthesiology, and gain a different perspective of cardiopulmonary resuscitation (CPR).
- Part III focuses on navigating complex systems: how time affects decision making, why mistakes compound over time, and how every intervention has the potential to cause more harm than good. I will share my successes and failures in the operating room, lessons from my residency training, and why good intentions don't always yield good results.
- Part IV describes the characteristics of a well-managed com-

plex system: skin in the game, tail risks, and convexity. I will describe how personal liability, a healthy amount of paranoia, and investments in expertise create the best decision makers. Part IV also explores what happens when Black Swans become so rare that people don't believe they exist.

§ MY REASONS FOR WRITING THIS BOOK §

I wrote this book for four reasons:

- First, I want people to see anesthesiology the way I observed John's management in the ICU. From an outside perspective, anesthesiology is tedious, technical, and repetitive. From my perspective in the operating room, it is less routine than it seems and more extraordinary than it appears.
- Second, I want to show you how anesthesiology principles can be applied outside of the operating room to safeguard our most precious societal institutions and personal assets. If you feel the current management of political, social, or economic systems is out of touch with reality, then I invite you to continue reading. You will gain a deeper understanding of the synergistic systems that define our new uncertain world.
- Third, I want to describe how anesthesiologists developed their expertise. To become an anesthesiologist, one must complete four years of medical school, then four years of intense, immersive, structured apprenticeship called residency—named because newly minted physicians used to live in the hospital during their training. Today, doctors are a bit more "entitled," if you can call it that; our training is "limited" to only 80 hours a week. As a retired surgeon once told me, "The only problem with being on call every other night is I missed half the good cases!" The truth is, we all put in the long hours because we understand a minimum of eight years

of high-quality medical training is necessary to make high-quality medical decisions for our patients.

- Fourth, the future of anesthesiology is uncertain due to the replacement of physicians by nonphysician providers (NPPs) to maximize financial efficiency. The limited monetary benefits come at the expense of training new physicians. I want to document our wisdom before our culture of expertise is permanently damaged or destroyed.

By the end of the book, you will better understand Black Swans—from the cognitive processes of the human brain to the daily life or death moments in the operating room. You will see how *vigilance*, which means focused observation of potential complications, allows anesthesiologists to prevent Black Swans without knowing what they are or when they will occur. These "birds" are difficult to find because they appear only when we aren't looking for them. In our new world defined by uncertainty, we must keep our senses sharp and minds open. Seeing Black Swans requires both vigilance and creativity. Let the hunt begin!

PART I

Recognizing and Responding to Uncertainty

CHAPTER 1

Our Limited Perspective

"The core predicament of medicine—the thing that makes being a patient so wrenching, being a doctor so difficult, and being a part of society that pays the bills they run up so vexing—is uncertainty. With all that we know nowadays about people and diseases and how to diagnose and treat them, it can be hard to see this, hard to grasp how deeply uncertainty runs. As a doctor, you come to find, however, that the struggle in caring for people is more often with what you do not know than what you do. Medicine's ground state is uncertainty. And wisdom—for both the patients and doctors—is defined by how one copes with it."

—Dr. Atul Gawande

"Medieval man was a cog in a wheel he did not understand; modern man is a cog in a complicated system he thinks he understands."

—Nassim Taleb

Dutch explorer Willem de Vlamingh is generally credited with the first sighting of a black swan on January 12, 1697. After he sailed up an Australian river in what is now the city of Perth, he came to a large island in the middle of the river. The river was later named Swan River, and the island, now called Heirisson Island, is a popular tourist attraction. There is even a sculpture of De Vlamingh and a black swan along the shore of Swan River near the island. In order to find our Black Swans, we must take a different kind of voyage into our own cognition—the background machinery that creates our individual perceptions.[5]

Why is this voyage important? In order to safeguard our future, we first need to learn why Black Swans occur. What we will find is that our perception is divided into two different structures based on whether synergy is present. A simple system is a model without synergy, and a complex system is a model with synergy. As our world becomes more intertwined, the complex system, which includes Black Swans, becomes more common.

§ WHAT DO YOU MEAN YOU DON'T KNOW? §

During my third year of residency, I was rotating in the cardiac surgical intensive care unit (CSICU) when I was asked to admit a post-operative liver transplant patient. The request was strange for a few reasons: this particular transplant lasted 28 hours (8–14 is normal), liver transplant patients usually go to the surgical ICU, and the patient was on four presser medications to improve his blood pressure. When he arrived in the CSICU, both his abdomen and chest were covered in plastic because they were left open; sometimes surgeons choose not to close their incision if there is high risk of bleeding or additional surgical exploration. I could see his heart beating underneath the millimeter-thin orange

---

5   The sculpture is located in Burswood Park between Camfield Drive and the Swan River. It is called *Willem de Vlamingh*. A brief summary of his discovery can be found at lifeonperth. com, a website about the history of Perth, Australia. De Vlamingh is generally credited with the initial black swan sighting in Australia in 1697, even though English explorers also brought black swans back to England from Australia.

plastic. Two tubes protruded from his chest going to an extra-corporeal membrane oxygenation (ECMO) machine. ECMO is an external heart-lung machine utilized when the heart or lungs unexpectedly fail.

In the operating room, the patient had developed a blood clot that traveled to his heart and caused it to fail. Cardiothoracic surgeons were called for an emergent sternotomy, a procedure in which the breastbone is divided with a saw in order to perform surgery inside the chest. He was then connected to an ECMO machine, which takes deoxygenated blood from the right atrium, oxygenates it, then pumps it into the aorta followed by the rest of his body.

After ECMO, the liver transplant was performed. The patient's chest and abdomen were bleeding too much to close the incision, so the abdominal and chest incisions were left open with sterile plastic stapled over the skin. He was bleeding so much he required about 1.2 L of blood products per hour. Unfortunately, his brain had been without oxygen for too long in the operating room before ECMO. He was pronounced brain dead in the CSICU 36 hours later.

Thousands of livers are successfully transplanted every year, so why did this man have such a horrible complication? Early that morning, at 4:00 a.m., I explained the situation to his daughter. How do you tell someone you did everything right, but their father was still dead?

Sometimes in medicine, poor outcomes occur for no discernable reason, even when doctors do everything right. During my first year of residency, I was rotating on the general surgery service. We had a healthy, 44-year-old gentleman who developed an infection of his colon called diverticulitis. The colon wall eventually developed a hole, then bacteria spilled into his abdomen. Free bacteria in the abdomen is a life-threatening condition called peritonitis.

I helped operate on him in the middle of the night, removing his diseased section of colon and creating a colostomy. A colostomy is a hole in the large bowel sutured to the skin. It allows fecal matter to exit the body before contacting the diseased section of colon. After the colon heals, the colostomy is reversed, usually a few months later. He recovered uneventfully until post-operative day five when he developed worsening abdominal pain. I examined his chest and abdomen, finally arriving at his colostomy. It was black and dead.

We took him back to the operating room, resected 15 cm of dead colon, and then made a new colostomy. He recovered and left the hospital one week later without further complications. I will never forget the way the patient looked at my attending after that. I could tell he didn't fully trust him anymore. My attending had done everything right, but we still had a poor outcome. Worse still, we couldn't tell the patient why it happened.[6]

Later that month, my senior resident presented the colostomy case to the entire surgery department to see if his complication could have been avoided. After everyone reviewed the operative technique and post-operative management, they agreed the patient

---

6   In teaching hospitals, fully licensed physicians called "attending physicians" lead teams of medical students and resident physicians. "Attending" means a physician who has completed medical school, residency, and passed his or her final board exams. The attending teaches trainees on rounds, delegates tasks to them in a safe manner consistent with their level of training, and makes all final decisions concerning patient care. Residents and medical students rotate through different medical specialties as they progress through their training. They are always supervised by an attending. Fellowship is an optional one to three years of subspecialty training completed after residency. All fellows are fully trained physicians. They are still supervised by attendings but tend to have more autonomy.

had received the best care possible. The most senior colorectal surgeon said he had seen this strange sequence of events only one other time 30 years ago. His eyes softened for a brief second and he said, "It just happens sometimes. Don't take it personally." This was from a surgeon who had created and managed more colostomies than anyone in the hospital and probably the country. I breathed a little easier leaving that meeting, but I still didn't have an answer.

For a physician, there is no greater shame than to be distrusted by your patient. Anesthesiologists and surgeons understand surgery is very dangerous—they must perform at the highest level for the chance of success. But this felt different. What do you do when you perform at the highest level and you still fail? How do you not take it personally?

In the Introduction, we established complications occur most often in situations of high complexity because high complexity means high synergy, and high synergy means more Black Swans. It then makes sense why medical Black Swans (complications) occur more in highly complex patients. Complications occur because doctors cannot know everything. Our knowledge is limited by the human narrative, a first-person perspective within objective reality.

§ THE SNOW GLOBE EFFECT §

Consider a thought experiment I call *The Snow Globe Exercise*. Imagine you are inside a Snow Globe on a desk in a windowless Manhattan office building. When you look up, you see the office ceiling. To you, that is the limit of reality. Now imagine you punch through the Snow Globe and end up on the office desk. You realize the Snow Globe was not reality; it was just the limit of your perspective. You open the door to the office and realize there's a whole office building too. Now the building is the limit of your perspective. Then you walk outside, see New York City, and then the sky for the first time. Now the sky is the limit of your perspective. Then you launch into space, outside of the Snow Globe of Earth, and you see Earth itself is a giant Snow Globe. Taken one step further: what do you think our whole universe would look like if you could move beyond it and look back?

The two patient complications described above are examples of The Snow Globe Effect. Our understanding of medical complications is limited by our understanding of medicine. Perhaps one day, doctors will know why the blood clot occurred or the colostomy failed. At the time, we had no way to predict these two patients would have these complications. Even though we did everything right, the complications were unavoidable.

The true problem is, humans have an incomplete first-person perspective of objective reality. Cognitive psychologist Daniel Kahneman, who was awarded the 2002 Nobel Prize in Economics for his work on decision making during uncertainty, calls the perspective problem "what you see is all there is" (WYSIATI). His research suggests the human mind overemphasizes possibilities inside its perspective while underemphasizing possibilities outside of its perspective.[7]

It makes sense, doesn't it? The sky would seem like an unlikely possibility to someone who has never been outside a windowless Manhattan office. Because objective reality is the sum of all interactions, including those we can't perceive, our perception will always be imperfect. The difference between our perceptions and objective reality causes *perception blindness*, which is the discrep-

---

7   My conceptual link between WYSIATI and The Snow Globe Effect can be seen in Chapter 7 of
     Kahneman's book *Thinking, Fast and Slow*.

ancy between what we think should happen and what actually happens.

We will always have perception blindness, but the level of our blindness (and sight) can change. This is how medical mysteries of the past eventually become the science of the future. An interesting example of this can be found in the life of Franklin Delano Roosevelt (FDR), the 32nd president of the United States.

In the 1940s, high blood pressure was considered to be essential to human life due to improved blood flow to organs. That's why it is still called essential hypertension to this day. A normal blood pressure is 120/80 mmHg. FDR's blood pressure was well above 200/120. In fact, it was above 300/120 mmHg on the day he suffered a brain bleed and died. He was only 63 years old. Today, every doctor knows uncontrolled high blood pressure will lead to life-threatening complications, such as heart attack, stroke, and kidney failure.

What changed? Clearer perception and, in turn, better results. Improved understanding of high blood pressure now prevents countless complications every year. Cardiovascular research allowed doctors to break through their essential hypertension Snow Globe. If you told a physician from the 1940s high blood pressure was harmful, they would have laughed at you. After 75 years of cardiovascular research, things have clearly changed. Still, we don't accuse FDR's cardiologist of malpractice because there was no way for him to have known this link in the 1940s.[8]

Black Swans are complications that occur due to perception

---

8 FDR's dangerously high blood pressure is well documented. A summary of his medical treatment can be found in "Hypertensive Therapy: Attacking the Renin-Angiotensin System" by Dr. Timothy Bishop and Dr. Vincent M. Figueredo.

blindness. As our perceptions diverge from objective reality, we experience more Black Swans because our interactions with objective reality are based on a flawed understanding of it. Complications are "unexpected" because our first-person perspective limits our predictive ability. Furthermore, they are "explainable later in time" because dangerous situations seem "obvious" only after a complication occurs. Hindsight is 20/20. If you record every instance of the same dangerous situation, the randomness of Black Swans reveals itself.

§ SIMPLE AND COMPLEX SYSTEMS §

We can further understand perception blindness and Black Swans by defining simple and complex systems. A *simple system* assumes perception blindness does not exist; it is a $1 + 1 = 2$ model of reality. Every action has a defined effect solely attributable to the original action. A *complex system* is a $1 + 1 = 3$ model; the mathematical discrepancy accounts for Black Swans due to our inherently limited perspective.

A complex system is an organic structure of components that communicates with one another and responds to changes in real time. Complex systems are all around us. Common examples include the human body, the stock market, a class of fourth graders, or Los Angeles traffic. The interactions of individual components ultimately produce an effect greater than the sum of their separate effects. This is called synergy.

Complex systems exhibit synergy for three reasons: first, the components of a complex system can react to forecasts of their future (e.g., stock market predictions can cause future price changes that wouldn't have occurred without the prediction); second, the components can behave in unforeseen ways (e.g., medical complications, like the blood clot or black colostomy); third, the number of possible outcomes becomes unmanageably large as complex systems grow (e.g., people interacting on the streets of New York City). When complex systems have an excessive amount of synergy, they generate new ideas and innovations but also create Black Swans.

Conversely, simple systems—such as a math equation—are unchanging patterns describing *part* of a complex system. Simple systems are different from complex systems because they cannot react to predictions, they produce predictable results, and they follow the same rules regardless of size. The simple systems that form a complex system can describe only individual parts of the complex system, but the sum of the simple systems cannot predict the outcome of the complex system. Again, in a simple system, 1 + 1 = 2, but in a complex system, 1 + 1 = 3.

Let's model the simple system (pure cause and effect) and the complex system (dominated by synergy and Black Swans).

A general formula for objective reality is Individual Actions + Synergistic Interactions = Defined Effects + Synergistic Events. When synergy is small, synergistic events are functionally absent, so the formula becomes Actions + Synergistic Interactions = Defined Effects (1 + 1 = 2). In medicine, this looks like a young, healthy person going for a low-risk outpatient surgery. The chance of synergistic events, such as necrotic colostomy or blood clot, is functionally zero.

When synergy is high, outcomes do not resemble the original interaction. Instead, they resemble random synergistic complications. Any anesthesiologist or surgeon will tell you, complications occur more often in complex situations, such as when patients take multiple medications, have unknown medical histories, and experience life-threatening emergencies. This was my sick liver transplant or colostomy patient. Then, when synergy becomes very large compared to the defined effects of individual actions, the equation becomes Actions + Synergistic Interactions = Synergistic Events ($1 + 1 = 3$).

§ BETWEEN TWO WORLDS §

We've established synergy exists and drives complex system outcomes. Remember, in the simple system ($1 + 1 = 2$), synergy and Black Swans do not exist, but in the complex system, synergy is so high that the system acts like a random event generator; its outcomes are always Black Swans. Let's look at what those two worlds look like, keeping in mind our true reality is somewhere in the middle.

In the simple system, where Black Swans do not exist, the probability of an event occurring is proportional to the most common event. This can be modeled as a gaussian distribution, aka the normal curve. The normal curve is a statistical model used to describe the distribution of physical quantities found in nature.

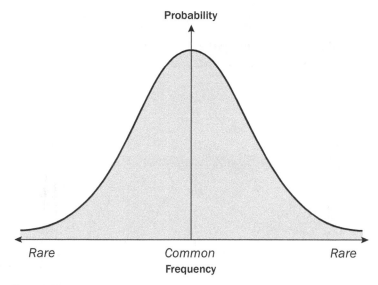

Figure 1-1

The X-axis is how often the event occurs, and the Y-axis is the probability of the event occurring. The further an event is from the average, the less chance it has of happening. Therefore, rare events have a small effect on the average because their size is inversely proportional to the chance of them occurring. Unreasonably large events have an unreasonably small probability of happening, so Black Swans are absent.

Common events have the largest effect because they occur most often. The gaussian distribution is used widely in mathematics, statistics, and risk management. However, it is not representative of reality when synergy is high. As our world becomes more synergistic, synergy will become dominant as it is in a complex system.

For the complex system, we will again graph the frequency of the event on the X-axis and the probability of an event occurring on the Y-axis. The next figure represents a large complex system.

Black Swans are the rare events on the right and left sides of the distribution. Common events are functionally absent because every event is rare, unique, and unexpected.

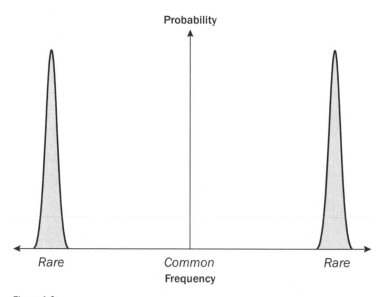

Figure 1-2

In complex systems, synergy increases much faster than the number of components. The relationship between the number of components and synergy is exponential. Therefore, as a number of part increases linearly, synergy increases infinitely. A complex system with infinite synergy is a random event generator. Their inputs will have no connection with their outputs. The outputs will only be Black Swans.

Below is a description of pure gaussian and pure synergistic worlds:[9]

9   My description of simple systems and complex systems is analogous to Nassim Taleb's
     Mediocrestan and Extremistan in his *Incerto*. My table is similar to Taleb's table in his book *The*
     Black Swan, Chapter 3, Table 1. I give him full credit for the idea.

GAUSSIAN WORLD	SYNERGISTIC WORLD
Dominated by a large number of small, common events	Dominated by a small number of large, rare events
Has no synergy	Only has synergy
Clear cause and effect	Random
Quantities with upper and lower limits	Quantities without limits
Usually physical, such as height	Usually numerical, such as money
Normal distribution of values	Only very large or very small values
Black Swans cannot exist	Only Black Swans exist

Figure 1-3

For example, money is a synergistic quantity and height is a gaussian quantity. Money grows without limit; height does not. The tallest person ever is about 5x taller than the shortest person ever and only 1.5x taller than the average person. However, the richest person in the United States is about 1,000,000x wealthier than the average African. In the United States, a billionaire is 10,000x richer than the average American. Synergistic quantities can be 100x, 1,000x, or even 100,000x larger than the average. Gaussian quantities are usually no more than 10x larger than the average. Gaussian models break down in the synergistic world because they do not account for large outliers that have a disproportionally large effect on the system.[10]

§ ABSENCE OF EVIDENCE IS NOT EVIDENCE OF ABSENCE §

In one world, cause and effect are discernable; in the other, cause and effect does not exist. As our world becomes more synergistic, the unknowable part will become a larger part of objective real-

---

10 Taken from worlddata.info/average-income.php. Specific numbers may differ, but orders of magnitude estimation are likely the same.

ity. Our true reality lies somewhere between the two theoretical extremes:

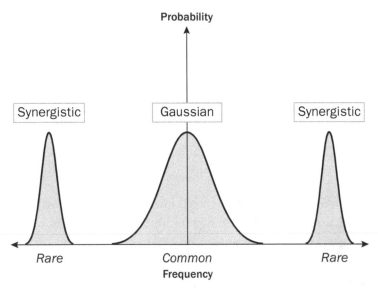

Figure 1-4

Humans easily conceptualize cause and effect, but synergy is more abstract. We need a different way to think about synergistic interactions so we can manage synergy appropriately. Blaming an individual for a synergistic Black Swan will not solve the problem because Black Swans are not caused by individual actions. They are caused by individual actions recombining in unpredictable ways.

Complex systems have immense practical value because they accurately model synergistic interactions and Black Swans. When the problems can be modeled, they can be studied, and when they can be studied, solutions can be found. I am writing through the lens of anesthesiology not only because I am an anesthesiologist but because anesthesiologists are already experts in the management of complex systems.

Anesthesiologists learned to study undesirable synergy, measure it, then extinguish it before it organizes into a Black Swan. We reported negative synergistic events (Black Swans), then systematically studied the synergistic factors associated with the event. Over the course of decades, patterns emerged, new strategies were tested, and results were restudied. This strategy, integrated over the last 70 years, changed anesthesiology into the reliable, consistent system we have today.

Overall, patients are older, sicker, and have more advanced medical problems than ever before in history, but anesthesiologists are still one step ahead, recognizing and treating complications before they organize into Black Swans. Anesthesia appears as a simple system because anesthesiologists manage the complex component of it. We understand how to control complexity to the extent it appears not to exist.

In recent history, our world has become more synergistic, but it is still treated like a pure simple system. This is problematic because simple and complex systems are fundamentally different. Simple systems can only grow to a maximum size, whereas complex systems grow to an infinite size, then if not maintained properly, will produce catastrophic Black Swans. Left on their own, they will destroy the system (or people) who created them.

So what hope is left? If Black Swans and complex systems are by definition unpredictable, how can we know how to manage them? The key is understanding how to think about uncertainty, synergy, and Black Swans. For anesthesiologists, that process takes four years of an undergraduate degree followed by four years of medical school, followed by four years of residency. Thankfully, we can glean quite a bit of wisdom from the time anesthesiologists have already invested. We'll start in medical school by meeting Dr. Charles Lucas and Dr. Anna Ledgerwood.

CHAPTER 2

Expertise, a Solution

"To study the phenomenon of disease without books is to sail an uncharted sea, while to study books without patients is not to go to sea at all."

—Dr. William Osler

"There is a big difference between getting experience and becoming an expert. The difference lies in the ability to identify when the outcomes of our decisions have something to teach us and what the lesson might be."

—Annie Duke, Professional Poker Player

When I applied to medical school in 2012, the three best known medical schools in Michigan were Wayne State in Detroit, University of Michigan in Ann Arbor, and Michigan State in Lansing. After I started my medical education at Wayne State, I heard a curious anecdote about my school's philosophy toward medical education:

> Three medical students arrive at the bedside of a critically ill patient. Their attending physician asks them what should be done. The first medical student from Michigan State is still

talking to the patient about his life. The second medical student from University of Michigan can recite the most up-to-date research but has no idea what to do. And the third medical student from Wayne State has no idea what is wrong with the patient but knows exactly what to do about it.

The point of the story is to emphasize Wayne State's philosophy of medical education rather than put down the University of Michigan or Michigan State. Wayne State's philosophy of medical education emphasizes experiential learning. The three medical students from the story represent the three things required for true expertise: knowledge (University of Michigan), metacognition (Michigan State), and experience (Wayne State).[11]

In this chapter, we'll explore the reasons physicians are considered experts. For the purpose of this book, I define expert as "a person who, over the course of many years, accumulates knowledge, metacognition, and experience that enables him or her to make consistent accurate predictions in uncertain real-life situations." True experts possess an expanded perspective enabling them to successfully navigate uncertainty.

§ LUCAS AND LEDGERWOOD §

I began to understand expertise as a medical student during my trauma surgery rotation when I met Dr. Charles Lucas and Dr. Anna Ledgerwood.

Dr. Ledgerwood has a powerful personality. Don't let her innocent-looking tuft of white hair or Midwest accent fool you.

---

11 Many theories of knowledge and models of expertise exist. Mine describes how physicians think about uncertainty. It might serve the practical purpose of defining who is credible based on their ability to interpret uncertainty.

She trained in an era when women traditionally did not become surgeons, so she had to work twice as hard to get half as much as her male counterparts. Her mind has only become sharper with age. When she walks into a room, everyone knows who is in charge. Dr. Ledgerwood expects her residents and medical students to perform at her level whether they like it or not. Her green eyes can read your thoughts before you speak. Her kindness is as boundless as her anger. She will hug her patient one minute and erupt at her residents the next.

Dr. Lucas has a different style. He's tall and thin with pale blue-gray eyes and walks slowly with his hands comfortably folded behind his lower back. He can communicate complex thoughts with a single look. He's the kind of person who doesn't speak many words, but when he does, everyone listens. Dr. Lucas has a different effect on his trainees. Even though you might meet him only a few times in your training, he feels like your most trusted mentor. He is the father figure you never knew you had.

With Dr. Ledgerwood, you fear her wrath; with Dr. Lucas, you fear his disappointment. I remember watching him examine a patient before taking her into the operating room. When she shuddered at his touch, he moved his right hand to his chest, produced a rare smile, and said, "Cold hands, warm heart." And that was all the patient needed to know she'd be okay.

Rounds with "the Ls" were quite different from other rotations. My first time rounding with Dr. Ledgerwood, she was appalled I didn't know where my patient went to high school. Medical students are expected to be encyclopedias of their patients, but I was still surprised by her level of expectation. From that day forward, I knew I had to buckle up and brace myself. My schedule was as follows: read the night before about my patients' pathologies, arrive at the hospital at 5:30 a.m., prepare my presentation for rounds, and then be "pimped" during rounds by Dr. Ledgerwood.[12]

If I didn't know the answer within five seconds, I was in trouble. Dr. Ledgerwood would then ask the residents detailed questions about pathophysiology. The best medical students could answer all of her questions, so the residents could relax in the background. If our whole team didn't know the answer, Dr. Ledgerwood would yell, "THIS PATIENT NEEDS A DOCTOR! ARE YOU THAT DOCTOR? ARE YOU THAT DOCTOR? BECAUSE RIGHT NOW, I DON'T SEE ANY DOCTORS!" She looked us in the eyes individually as she'd say this, and when she felt especially offended, she would turn around and walk away in disgust.

Rounds with Dr. Ledgerwood was intense-intense, whereas rounds with Dr. Lucas were calm-intense. When medical students didn't know the answers to his questions, Dr. Lucas would sigh, look down at his feet, and shake his head. The sense of disappointment was overwhelming, especially because we knew he wouldn't let us finish our presentation. Instead, he'd ask the chief resident to summarize the rest and move on.

After rounds, I spent the rest of my day assisting in the operating room or carrying out tasks for recovering patients on the surgical ward. My job was to be helpful in any way possible: from holding a retractor for hours in the operating room to faxing paperwork. Of course, I also wanted to learn from my patients. I remember many of their cases with great detail.

12　"Pimping" is the Socratic method applied in medical education. The Socratic method is a form of cooperative argument where both parties stimulate critical thinking in the other. In medical education, attendings ask medical students and residents about their fund of knowledge and thinking process to expose gaps in their knowledge or flaws in their reasoning. The trainees try to make their attending run out of questions. It's like psychological chess.

One of them was a dangerously thin, elderly African American man with a short beard streaked with gray. His eyes were deep and brown as though they had endured a difficult life. I saw him in the emergency room because he was coughing up blood. He had a distinct black, shiny, foul-smelling stool called melena, which suggested a bleed in the esophagus or stomach. I passed a nasogastric tube into his nose, past his palate, arriving in his stomach. Immediately, 500 cc of blood was suctioned out. He was then admitted to our general surgery service for management of a presumed stomach bleed.

Over the next day, he received blood transfusions and an endoscopic exam of his stomach. His stomach biopsy showed a rare tumor called gastric MALToma, a cancer of the lymphatic tissue in the stomach wall. This cancer is usually caused by a bacterial infection called *Helicobacter pylori* and is the only cancer that can be treated with antibiotics in the early stages. In this case, the cancer was eroding the wall of the stomach but had not metastasized. He would require radiation and possibly chemotherapy in addition to antibiotics.

During his five-day hospital admission, we walked laps together in the ward hallway every day. I learned everything about his medical history, histology, pathophysiology, cancer staging, chemotherapy, radiation, and eligible clinical trials. I also learned about him as a person: his strained relationship with his family, past heroin use, intermittent homelessness, and how he slept in an abandoned attic for the last month.

On the last day of my rotation, I was rounding with Dr. Ledgerwood. This time, I knew everything about my patient, including his medical history, social history, treatment options for his stomach cancer, and where he would go after discharge. Despite the fact I spent three hours preparing the night before, my presentation lasted a mere two minutes. After I answered all of her questions, her eyes narrowed, she huffed air from her nose, and then stormed off without another word. As soon as she turned the corner, I danced in the hallway. I had received the highest compliment a third-year medical student on her service could receive: her lack of criticism.

With Dr. Lucas and Dr. Ledgerwood, I learned expertise is built on a foundation of knowledge. Experts can't know they are correct unless they have a comprehensive knowledge of their subject. Missing a single detail could be the difference between life and death. This lesson would be confirmed over and over again in my anesthesiology residency training.

§ KNOWLEDGE §

Medical students are knowledge sponges. Every three months of medical school is approximately one undergraduate science degree (120 undergraduate credit hours). After two years of book learning, students take an eight-hour cumulative exam. Then in the third year of medical school, students rotate in different specialties. They are tested once per month on their clinical knowledge. After third year, they take another eight-hour cumulative exam. The overwhelming amount of knowledge acquired in medical school is commonly described as "drinking from a fire hose." For perspective, I learned an entire semester of undergraduate immunology in 12 days.[13]

Knowledge is the first component of expertise. To become a true

---

13   These cumulative exams are called USMLE (United States Medical Licensing Exam) STEP 1 and STEP 2. The amount of material covered is approximately 5,000 textbook pages each. Learning how to memorize, then organize this volume of information is a skill in itself.

expert, one must divide their knowledge into three layers: things they know, things they know they don't know, and things they don't know they don't know. A diagram of this three-layer model is shown below.

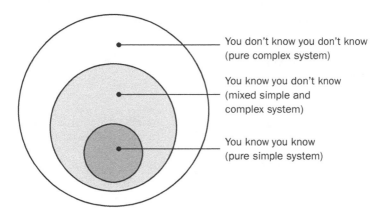

You don't know you don't know
(pure complex system)

You know you don't know
(mixed simple and
complex system)

You know you know
(pure simple system)

Figure 2-1

The following are diagrams for a medical student (start of training), resident (middle of training), and attending (fully trained).

MEDICAL STUDENT

You don't know you don't know
(pure complex system)

Figure 2-2

Medical students should know every fact about their patients because they don't know what is important. One of my attendings once told me, "Ask all your questions as a medical student because you won't have time to ask them in residency." To a medical student, the world appears as a large complex system (random event generator). They are always surprised—ask me how I know!

RESIDENT

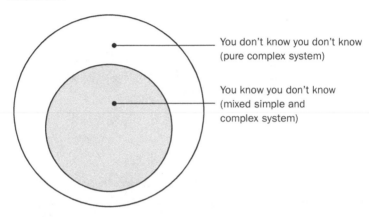

You don't know you don't know
(pure complex system)

You know you don't know
(mixed simple and
complex system)

Figure 2-3

To residents, the world is a complex system that includes some cause and effect. They are trained to be cautious, especially when encountering new situations, so they don't cause preventable complications. There is always an attending physician immediately available just in case. That same attending also told me, "Make all your mistakes as a resident because you will have no one to correct them when you are an attending." Residents are usually frustrated because this learning occurs through years of tedious trial and error with an attending constantly micromanaging you— ask me how I know!

ATTENDING

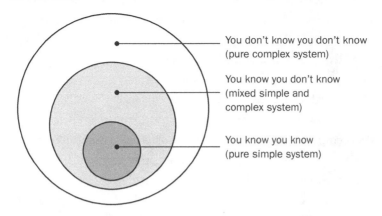

You don't know you don't know
(pure complex system)

You know you don't know
(mixed simple and
complex system)

You know you know
(pure simple system)

Figure 2-4

Attendings have all three layers and can differentiate between them. They know when they are comfortable with a situation (first layer), when they are capable but need to be extra focused or acquire additional attainable knowledge (second layer), and when they do not have the expertise to properly evaluate a situation (third layer). At this point, they might consult another expert. No physician is an expert in everything, but they know what they don't know. True experts understand the limits of their knowledge because they can accurately triage data into the three layers, then give an informed opinion about how external data relates to their internal knowledge.

Physicians must also learn how to weigh different kinds of knowledge. Subjective knowledge exists in the mind of an individual—it may or may not exist in objective reality because it consists of one person's limited perspective. Objective knowledge exists regardless of perception. Some examples of objective knowledge are bacteria, the sun, and gravity. They are independent of human perspective—that is, if all humans became extinct tomorrow, they would still exist. Bacteria existed before humans could see them with microscopes. The sun existed before humans existed. Gravity works whether you believe in it or not. Subjective knowledge exists in the fallible perspective of a single individual; objective knowledge can be observed independent of individual perspective.

The crucial difference between the two allows physicians to separate knowledge into the three layers. Doctors even structure their communication in terms of subjective and objective quantities. Unmeasurable quantities (subjective knowledge) include the patient's perspective of his or her suffering and the physician's perspective of the patient. Measurable quantities (objective knowledge) include the physical exam, labs, and imaging studies. We weigh each factor differently depending on the individual situation. Diagnosis is not following an algorithm. We need to see thousands of patients in a variety of clinical scenarios before we develop expert-level judgment.

§ METACOGNITION §

Dr. Lucas and Dr. Ledgerwood were correct to treat me with healthy suspicion. Even with the proper knowledge, medical students initially struggle to understand *which* knowledge is most relevant. Rounds help medical students organize their knowledge into subjective and objective components. This process is called metacognition, defined as "thinking about thinking." Metacognition, the second element of expertise, is the mechanism by which experts arrange knowledge into the three layers.

This process requires abstraction, which is the transformation of unrelated things into a common idea. Abstraction is a metacognitive language that allows humans to quickly communicate relationships between objects. Similes and metaphors are common examples. A boat is to the water as a car is to the...? (Road). A boat could be called a water car, just as a car could be called a road boat. Both are different objects but share the abstract quality of transportation. Abstraction can be separated into intelligence (abstraction with facts) and empathy (abstraction with feelings).

Intelligence is the measure of how well an individual reconciles their individual perspective with objective reality. For medical students, this is measured by standardized tests and clinical performance. We must reconcile our imprecise perceptions with the objective anatomy, physiology, and pathology of our patients. Those who can adapt their perception to an external set of facts and/or patterns are typically considered intelligent. Examples include an engineer designing a machine consistent with the laws of physics, a poet writing poetry consistent with the existential conflicts of human nature, or a medical student diagnosing disease consistent with his or her patient's symptoms, physical exam, labs, and imaging.

Empathy is abstraction relating human feelings. It allows us to recognize other humans as an extension of ourselves. Humans tend to become upset after hurting someone else unintentionally because we recognize the pain they feel as our own pain. Abstraction with feelings allows us to communicate patterns of relationships across a wide variety of experiences. For example, the Greeks had six words for "love" describing different ways people could be empathetically related. *Agape* means seeking the best for others regardless of circumstance, *eros* means romantic love, *philia* means friendship, *storge* is affection between parents and their children, *philautia* is loving oneself, and *xenia* means reciprocal hospitality between hosts and travelers. Expertise is by definition a human creation and therefore only exists in the context of human relationships.

Dr. Lucas and Dr. Ledgerwood taught empathy in unique ways. I especially remember how Dr. Ledgerwood would make us present her patients during rounds. Before rounds started at 6:30 a.m., we had to get our patients out of bed, sit them up in a chair, and place a clean white bedsheet folded in half in their lap. Their hospital gown and face needed to be clean. If her patients were not perfectly presented, she would accuse us of not caring about them and question our motives as doctors. After aggressively testing us for intellectual abstraction during rounds, she would walk into each patient's room and treat them as her own family. She would sit next to them and talk with them about their feelings, their fears, and their future. She wanted her trainees to recognize their humanity in their patients.

Another one of my memorable patients was an exceedingly pleasant African American man in his 70s. I ended up meeting him because his wife forced him to see a doctor after he saw blood in his urine. The workup included a CT scan of his abdomen, which revealed a cancer in his right colon. Luckily for him, the cancer had not spread to the rest of his body yet. The thing I remember most about this man was his smile. He was kind to everyone around him no matter what happened. He had a bald shiny head, and the only wrinkles on his face were at the corners of his eyes and lips, presumably from a lifetime of smiling.

When he was first admitted to the surgical ward, I took his history and examined him. As I asked him about his history, he quickly noticed my speech impediment. He told me he also had a stutter growing up. We spent an hour talking about how we overcame our difficulties: he read poetry out loud and I went to speech therapy. His wife and daughter were relieved he "finally went to the doctor after all these years." I quickly learned their patience had finally grown thin. Their family banter was a constant source of amusement.

After two days of planning, we took him to the operating room to remove his colon cancer. I assisted in the operation and even felt the edge of his liver for possible metastases. The edge was warm, soft, and smooth. It had the texture of cold butter and the temperature of warm bathwater. After his surgery, we walked laps around the surgical ward every day as he recovered.

I updated him and his family every day of his progress. I checked on him twice a day: once before rounds and once in the afternoon. When he left the hospital, our connection had grown. His wife, ever the pragmatist, told him to "stop being weird" as she gently wheeled him toward the elevator. Empathy had built trust, and trust had built a (student) doctor-patient relationship.

§ EXPERIENCE, FALSE EXPERTS, AND COMPLEXITY §

The third element of expertise is experience. Experience is essential for expertise because it validates knowledge and metacognition in objective reality. Obtaining knowledge and metacognition prior to practicing is helpful because it allows the expert to organize experiences into meaningful patterns rather than simply memorizing facts.

Practicing without a basic understanding of principles is like memorizing the sounds of words instead of learning how to read. The memorizer is not literate because he or she does not have the knowledge or metacognition to understand what he or she is reading. Unlike a literate person who can read an unlimited number of texts, the illiterate person can only copy what he or she memorized. The illiterate person cannot read because he or she doesn't understand the basic rules of literacy.

In medical education, we don't let medical students touch patients until they prove they have the knowledge and metacognitive literacy to do so safely. The preclinical years are for acquiring knowledge, the clinical years for metacognition, and residency is for experience. We need to see thousands of different patients in different settings in order to develop basic medical literacy. My final literacy test will be both written and oral exams administered by the American Board of Anesthesiology. If I pass, I can practice medicine unsupervised as a true expert.

True experts can organize their knowledge into three layers and differentiate between subjective and objective knowledge. Over time, their performance will improve because they can interpret and adapt to the world around them. Some examples include professional sports players, physicians, and mechanics.

False experts are people who claim to be an expert but do not meet the criteria of a true expert. They lack knowledge (do not know basic information), metacognition (cannot meaningfully organize their thoughts), experience (direct interaction with reality), or results (ability to make correct predictions in uncertain situations).

You can apply this standard to daily life to identify false experts and misinformation. False experts assume their individual perspective is a perfect representation of reality. They will resort to conspiracy thinking instead of acknowledging additional actions exist outside of their perspective. They will disagree with known experts about basic facts and claim to have an extensive fund of knowledge without evidence. Some will even claim to "do their own research" but lack the knowledge, metacognition, or experience to confirm their "expertise."

False experts often have difficulty differentiating between facts, inferences, and opinions. A fact can be proven beyond a reasonable doubt; it is objective knowledge. An example would be driving faster consumes more gasoline. Inferences are conclusions drawn from facts; they may or may not be true. They are a simple system with a complex component. An example would be driving faster consumes more gas; therefore, raising speed limits will increase smog. Opinions can be statements from personal, religious, or political ideologies that cannot be confirmed or refuted. They have nothing to do with analytical thought or a discussion of the truth. An example would be, "Cars are my favorite kind of transportation."

Finally, many problems of today's complex systems rest on a simple premise: those who declare themselves experts are not responsible for the results of their opinions. Lack of accountability for false predictions encourages people to rely on luck rather than skill.

False experts might make many vague predictions, hope one of them becomes true by luck alone, then claim they "knew it the whole time." This is equivalent to someone claiming they had a 100% shooting percentage after making only one of ten free throws. In the other nine instances, the person missed. True experts will be correct in the vast majority of their predictions even when their failures are counted.

After a significant amount of knowledge, metacognition, and experience accumulate, a true expert literally sees the world differently than nonexperts. Their expanded perspective can quickly triage complications others cannot even perceive. Physicians acquire this cognitive structure in medical school. In anesthesiology, I use it every day to manage unexpected events in the operating room and ICU. I'm grateful for Dr. Lucas's and Dr. Ledgerwood's example of expertise. Ultimately, they showed me how to correctly organize my mind in order to manage complexity and Black Swans.

This cognitive model might be applied outside of the operating room to other situations. Objectively defining our own level of expertise allows us to make better decisions about uncertainty. If we can better evaluate the limit of our knowledge, we can better predict when to trust our own opinions rather than following the advice of someone with more expertise. Knowledge, meta-cognition, and experience can be compared between individuals to figure out who is the best qualified to evaluate an uncertain situation.[14]

So far, we've seen how to recognize and classify synergistic inter-actions and how experts approach their learning to prepare for and respond to uncertainty. Next, we will explore the difference between productive and unproductive responses to uncertainty. Years of training are necessary to reprogram our brains to respond appropriately because our own psychology works against us. Here, we will see why experts need extensive experience to face the ever-increasing complexity in our world.

---

14 In order to have constructive interactions, we need to understand the limits of our knowledge. The old saying "The less you know, the more you think you know" is truer today than ever before in history. If we cannot define the limits of our expertise, we will have a society of false experts. If you lack expertise in a subject, your opinion in that subject area is highly likely to be incorrect. If you think you know more than an expert, you should articulate why your opinion is superior despite having less knowledge, metacognition, and experience.

CHAPTER 3

Finding Confidence in Complexity

"For a long time it had seemed to me that life was about to begin—real life. But there was always some obstacle in the way, something to be gotten through first, some unfinished business, time still to be served, a debt to be paid. Then life would begin. At last it dawned on me that these obstacles were my life."

—Alfred D'Souza

"Death does not wait for you to be ready! Death is not considerate or fair! And make no mistake: here, you face Death!"

—Henri Ducard, *Batman Begins*

The first year of residency training is called intern year. It includes a variety of clinical rotations designed to teach new medical school graduates how to apply their knowledge. Think of it as doctor boot camp. My intern year was composed of five months of surgery rotations (trauma, thoracic, colorectal, hepatobiliary, orthopaedics), three months of ICU (medical, surgical, neurosurgical), one month of emergency medicine, one month of neurology, one month of anesthesiology preoperative clinic, two weeks of internal medicine, and two weeks of anesthesiology in the operating room.

Intern year is the first time physicians experience the magnitude of their responsibilities. No amount of book learning can prepare you for holding a human life in your hands. Furthermore, the application of knowledge to a unique human being is fundamentally different than the academic patterns learned in medical school. Extensive experience in stressful, ambiguous situations refines and reorganizes our extensive knowledge and metacognition to function in complex domains.

There is no perfect way to approach the application of knowledge. Eventually, you have to jump into the deep end of the pool and start paddling: either you learn to swim or you drown.

§ JANUARY 1, 2018—FACING DEATH §

Six months into my intern year, I was on 24-hour trauma surgery call during New Year's Eve. The hospital was pandemonium. My pager went off so often I couldn't answer and delete my pages fast enough.[15]

In the emergency room, patients overflowed into the hallway; they were young, mostly intoxicated, and some were even wearing costumes. This was West Los Angeles after all. I sat down three times in 24 hours. Finally, at 5:30 a.m. the following day, I signed out to my fellow intern and turned off my pager. All I had to

---

15   Yes, physicians still use pagers. The main advantage over a cell phone is physicians can triage the messages as needed. Less urgent messages can wait while more urgent ones are taken care of. When I'm in the trauma bay, I can ignore the messages, then answer them when it's safe to do so. Pagers suffer fewer complications compared to cell phones, are cheaper to replace, and don't need software updates. Sometimes a simple device that can't fail is better than a more complex one prone to Black Swans.

do was round on my 12 colorectal surgery patients, write notes, and go home.

After I reviewed the morning labs and vitals, I received a call from one of the general surgery chief residents. The intern on call was taking care of a different emergency, so he requested my assistance in the trauma bay. Four patients involved in a horrific car accident were on their way to the emergency department. I dropped my list of colorectal patients and ran to the ED.

The four patients required every available physician and nurse. They were all in the same car hit by a drunk driver. All of them were in critical condition. The senior surgical resident managed the first two traumas himself, intubated both, and managed their triage—one went to the operating room and the other to the CT scanner. The junior surgical resident managed the third trauma, intubated him, and took him to the second available CT scanner. I managed the fourth trauma with an emergency medicine (EM) attending physician nearby.

After several minutes, the EM physician and I noticed our patient's decline in mental status, meaning he closed his eyes and became somnolent. This was concerning because it meant he might not be able to breathe on his own or "protect his airway." When someone loses consciousness, oral secretions and stomach contents can travel into the lungs causing a severe chemical inflammation called aspiration pneumonia. We both agreed the patient should have a breathing tube inserted to prevent both complications.

A few minutes later, two anesthetic drugs were injected, and then I was handed a direct laryngoscope to visualize the vocal cords. There are two kinds of laryngoscopy: direct and video. In direct laryngoscopy, the physician must move the tongue and epiglottis out of the way in order to create a straight line of sight to the vocal cords. In video laryngoscopy, a lens at the end of the laryngoscope blade displays the image on an external screen. Video laryngoscopy is easier because you don't need to move anatomic structures out of the way. The video camera does most of the work for you. The surgical residents used both of the video laryngoscopes, so I was left with a more difficult task.[16]

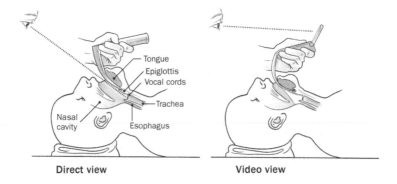

Direct view   Video view

Figure 3-1

Successful direct laryngoscopy relies on precise millimeter-sized movements of the elbow and shoulder. Small, accidental shifts can cause failure. As I felt the patient's jaw relax and his breathing stop, I slid the laryngoscope past the right side of the tongue. Just as I achieved an excellent view of the vocal cords, I heard a loud sound. For a split second, I looked to see what it was. When I looked back at the patient, I could only see tongue and throat. Not good.

---

16   Advantages of video laryngoscopy include improved glottic visualization, higher nonexpert success rate, less cervical spine manipulation, and less force necessary to obtain a view of the vocal cords. Disadvantages include difficulty in passing the endotracheal tube despite improved visualization, possible increased intubation time, variable learning curve, potential weakening of direct laryngoscopy skill, false confidence by nonexperts, and the lens can be obscured by oral secretions or blood. Currently, the American Society of Anesthesiologists lists video laryngoscopy as an adjunct to "Alternative Difficult Intubation Approaches." An excellent review article is "Videolaryngoscopy" by Dr. Raffi Chemsian, published in 2014.

Because he was fully anesthetized, he could no longer breathe on his own. His body was consuming the last of the oxygen in his blood. Oxygen saturation measures the amount of oxygen carried by red blood cells; normal values in a healthy person are >95%. Now my patient's oxygen saturation started to drop—first to 94, then 93, then 92, 91…I knew I had to get the tube in before his oxygen saturation dropped further…88, 86, 84…my heart rate skyrocketed…82, 80…

At this point, I was physically and mentally exhausted. I hadn't slept in over 24 hours. Then, in an instant, I experienced a brief moment of clarity. I slid the direct laryngoscope past the tongue, moved the epiglottis out of the way, achieved an excellent view of the vocal cords, then smoothly passed the endotracheal tube past the vocal cords. As I ventilated my patient with a purple AMBU bag, his saturation continued to drop. Then it bottomed out at 68%. Eventually, it slowly rose back to 100%. It felt like the slowest intubation of my life, but it probably lasted less than ten seconds.

In that moment, I felt like my sympathetic nervous system (fight-or-flight response) was turned off. Afterward, I checked my heart rate: it was exactly 60. One beat per second. I stayed with my patient in the CT scanner until the rest of the trauma team took over for me. I rounded on my colorectal patients, went home, slept for 16 hours, then woke up at 4:30 a.m. the following day. I arrived at the hospital before sunrise.

There comes a point where all young physicians must face the possibility of death alone and unaided. No one can teach you how to handle these circumstances. This point in my training marked a transition in how I approached uncertainty. I learned how to suppress my automatic response to stress so I could perform under the pressure of having another human life in my hands. This trait is essential for dealing with uncertainty.

Psychologically, humans crave black-and-white, simple narratives of the world. However, as our reality becomes more complex that simple narrative will occur less often. Black and white will become shades of gray. Therefore, it's best to train our nervous system to respond to the stress of uncertainty in a constructive rather than destructive manner. Let's now dive into how cognitive psychology explains this phenomenon.

§ SYSTEM 1 AND SYSTEM 2 §

In his book *Thinking, Fast and Slow*, Daniel Kahneman put forth an interesting model for these two ways of thinking. He called them System 1 and System 2. System 1 is fast, automatic, and emotional, whereas System 2 is slow, effortful, and logical. System 1 includes the fight-or-flight response I felt when I was distracted; System 2 is more analytical and detail oriented. Below is a table summarizing both systems of thinking:[17]

---

17   Descriptions of both systems were derived from Chapter 1 of *Thinking, Fast and Slow*. The systems are cognitive models that correspond to human decision-making patterns found in psychology experiments. They do not anatomically exist.

	SYSTEM 1	SYSTEM 2
CHARACTERISTICS	Fast, automatic, emotional, unconscious	Slow, effortful, logical, conscious
	Speaks before thinking	Thinks before speaking
	Evaluates Gestalt	Evaluates individual details
	Impulsive	Deliberate
WHAT DOES IT DO?	Localizes source of a sound	Searches memory for specific sound
	Completes simple sentences	Creates complex sentences
	Solves simple math problems	Solves multistep math problems
	Drives a car on an empty road	Drives a car in heavy traffic
WHEN IS IT USED?	Runs automatically in background	Must be consciously turned on
EXAMPLE	Karen or Smudge the Cat memes	Chess champion

Figure 3-2

The cognitive model of System 1 and System 2 explains the differences between my first and second attempts at intubation. During my first attempt, I was in System 1 focused on my exhaustion, fear, and anxiety. My second attempt was System 2: focused, deliberate, and calm. I somehow blocked out all other stimulation in the room so I could 100% focus on the intubation. During that moment, nothing else existed—only my hands, the laryngoscope, and the breathing tube.

I felt like a doctor for the first time. I also realized if I let my System 1 get the best of me, I could seriously hurt a patient. I was taught to remain calm in medical school, but I didn't truly understand it until a patient's life depended solely on my performance. No amount of knowledge or metacognition could help me in that moment.

Becoming a doctor meant I needed to default to System 2 rather than the automatic System 1. The second half of intern year, I saw every crisis, angry patient, and concerned nurse as an opportunity to push my cognition further into System 2. Instead of viewing intern year as a "rite of passage" or "hazing," I viewed it as an opportunity to develop my cognition.

I still arrived at the hospital before the sun rose and left after it set, but I saw the hospital in a different light. On my surgical ICU rotation, I saw the sun four times. I was still tired, hungry, and had to work long hours for minimal pay. I still struggled with sick patients, demanding nurses, and my own lack of experience. But I wasn't the same person anymore. The most basic mechanism underlying all of my cognition had permanently changed.

§ HEPATOBILIARY SURGERY—STAYING IN SYSTEM 2 §

Residency is not like it is portrayed on television. Most of the time, interns are so tired they would rather *sleep* than try to *sleep with* each other. For the entire year, I worked 12-plus-hour days six days per week writing notes, coordinating admissions, and organizing discharges. I was regularly on call for 28 hours at a time. When I was home, I read about my patients, their diseases, and surgeries so I wouldn't make a mistake the following day. I felt like I was constantly treading water. I could feel it splashing into my mouth, dangerously close to drowning in the volume of work and responsibility.[18]

The stress of intern year flowed into other aspects of my life. I moved to Los Angeles a week before starting residency. Unfor-

---

18 Thinking critically (and quickly) in emergencies is a skill that can only be learned through making decisions in critical situations. Residency is challenging on purpose so physicians develop this vital skill.

tunately, none of my belongings had arrived from Michigan. All I had was my backpack where I kept my wallet, computer, keys, and passport…Then I lost my backpack during my first week of intern year. I went to the office of Alan Pierce, one of the medical education administrators, and cried. Luckily, I found my backpack three days later in the eighth-floor operating room. Definitely a System 1 moment.

My most difficult rotation was hepatobiliary surgery. I managed 15 to 25 hepatobiliary surgical patients. I rounded on them, assisted in their operations, wrote daily progress notes, and eventually coordinated their discharges. Common reasons for surgery included pancreatic cancer, intestinal blockages, liver cancer, and complex gallbladder problems. Many of these patients had multiple medical problems in addition to their primary surgical problem. I had to understand everything about their underlying conditions, how and why those conditions were affected by the surgeries, and the postoperative implications of their altered anatomy and physiology.

My attending, Dr. Nissen, had a hectic schedule, including scheduled surgeries in the mornings, clinic in the afternoons, and liver transplants at night. He would fit inpatient rounds into his schedule when he could. I never knew when he would round with me, so I had to be ready at all times. He would call me and simply say, "Rounds in 15 minutes. I'm on my way." When he arrived, we walked once around the surgical ward as I presented each patient in one sustained breath. To move at his pace, I had to know every vital sign, lab, imaging result, and patient symptom within seconds of being asked. Like Dr. Lucas and Dr. Ledgerwood, Dr. Nissen's high expectations moved me one step closer to true expertise.

I had to utilize every moment of the day in order to work only

12 hours per day so I could study at night. I created macros so I could quickly collect vital signs and write notes, made detailed checklists of all my tasks, and rounded on my own multiple times per day to make sure I was always one step ahead. I also learned to preemptively coordinate discharges with social workers and case managers so bureaucracy wouldn't slow me down.[19]

In addition to the logistical challenges, there were also emotional challenges. One day, I remember signing out, ready to leave the hospital at 6:00 p.m. As I was about to turn off my pager, it went off. A recently admitted gentleman in his 60s wanted to talk about the prognosis of his metastatic colon cancer. That day, we told him he was not a surgical candidate, meaning his liver metastasis excluded him from a curative operation. He would die from his colon cancer eventually. His daughter just arrived at the hospital and wanted to talk about his options.

I made my way to his room on the surgical ward. I talked with him and his daughter for two hours. They shared their concerns, existential worries, family tensions, legal implications of death, and fear of abandonment.

I addressed their questions one at a time in the best way I could, promising to make several referrals, including palliative care. We talked about how hospice care focuses on his comfort and quality of life and that hospice patients generally live longer with better quality of life than those who do not receive hospice care. I choked back tears as he and his daughter cried together. At 8:30 p.m., I finally left the hospital. Before going

---

19   A macro is a computer shortcut where a short piece of code—or in this case, text—is automatically substituted for a more complex one. I made macros for progress notes, labs, and physical exams so I could write a complete, detailed progress note in about 60 seconds.

to bed, I reviewed the medical and surgical management of liver metastases.[20]

I was learning to see the chaotic events around me as opportunities rather than burdens. When my hepatobiliary surgery rotation ended, I felt conflicted. I felt relieved from the intense pressure and razor-thin margin of error, but I also felt sadness. For the first time, I had experienced the visceral pleasure of performing at the highest level and succeeding in the face of overwhelming uncertainty.

This kind of performance, the kind required to thrive in uncertainty, can only be achieved in System 2. I learned to actively suppress my automatic, subconscious, and oftentimes counterproductive responses to uncertainty. In its place, I developed a more constructive System 2. I'm glad I learned this lesson when I did because after my intern year, residency became more difficult.

§ ANESTHESIOLOGY AND THE TWO SYSTEMS §

After intern year, I started my three years of anesthesiology training. The learning curve in the operating room is definitely steeper than intern year. Patients became hypotensive (low blood pressure), bradycardic (low heart rate), and hypoxic (low oxygen saturation) for seemingly no reason. I lived in a state of constant fear, but now I finally knew how to suppress System 1 and prioritize System 2. Over the course of the next three years, I learned

---

20 Hospice and palliative care is widely misunderstood. It does not mean "we are giving up." It means, "we acknowledge the patient is likely to live less than six months. Therefore, we should make additional efforts to focus on their quality of life and give appropriate medical therapies in line with their values." If a patient lives longer than expected, he or she can discontinue hospice care if medically appropriate. A summary of hospice and palliative care can be found at the National Institute of Aging website: nia.nih.gov/health/what-are-palliative-care-and-hospice-care.

to think faster than ever before. I developed an awareness and reaction time that would make hepatobiliary surgery look like slow motion.

During my third year, I intubated a ten-year old with a bowel obstruction. She would not breathe any oxygen before intubation and would not let us touch her IV. After we finally injected her with anesthetics, her altered physiology from the bowel obstruction in addition to her high heart rate caused her oxygen saturation to quickly to fall from 100% to 60% in 15 seconds. I intubated her in a fast, fluid motion without hesitation. In that moment, I remembered my New Year's Eve intubation. I had come a long way.

Anesthesiologists need to perform at the highest level because our world is a daily dance with death. Although most healthcare professionals become more frantic in emergencies, due to our training anesthesiologists become calmer. Our System 2 becomes faster than our System 1. We're able to remain in a state of internal focus no matter what is happening around us.

Events like hypoxia, bradycardia, and hypotension can cause death within minutes. We assume complications will occur, think statistically about their probability, then adjust our actions accordingly. A single overlooked detail can kill a patient. We need to thrive even in the most uncertain, critical situations.

EFFECT OF TRAINING ON ANESTHESIOLOGIST COGNITION

	SYSTEM 1	SYSTEM 2	COGNITION
MEDICAL STUDENT/INTERN	Dominant	Developing, inefficient	Nervous, not confident about even simple decisions, fears accidentally harming patients
RESIDENT	Becomes less prominent	Becomes more prominent	Confident yet hesitant, understands basic risks and benefits, acts decisively but doesn't always make the correct decision
ATTENDING	Fades into background	Dominant	Performs at highest level in uncertain and emergent situations, full cognitive homeostasis

Figure 3-3

During my fourth year of residency, I was called to emergently intubate a 100-year-old Persian gentleman who fell out of bed and broke his neck. His neck was supported in a hard cervical collar. His oxygen saturation was slowly decreasing, dropping 1% every 15 seconds. To make matters worse, he had a long list of medical problems, but no one knew any details about them.

I assertively called for a fiberoptic bronchoscope, a two-foot-long, flexible, black tube with a camera at the end. Successful fiberoptic intubation requires maneuvering around the delicate anatomy of the mouth and throat. Any injury to the mucosa can cause permanent damage, bleeding, and swelling and can make further intubation difficult or impossible.

As the nurses were getting the scope, I tried to put a sealed oxygen mask on the patient's face so I could assist his natural breathing with an AMBU bag. Because he was resisting us and in a hard collar, we were losing the battle. His oxygen saturation slowly drifted down to 70%. Finally, the fiberoptic scope arrived and was plugged into a portable monitor. I threaded a breathing tube over the fiberoptic scope, then prepared to guide the scope into his trachea. Then the monitor went black.

Two nurses quickly scurried away to find another monitor. Now I was in a difficult situation. If I took off his collar, I risked damaging his cervical spinal cord and causing quadriparesis (paralysis of all four limbs). His saturation continued to drift down to 60%. But there was another problem: giving him anesthetic medication would be very risky because he had a history of congestive heart failure, and no one knew how severe it was. In his fragile state, even small amounts of anesthetic medications could stop his heart.

Now his oxygen saturation was at 50%. I spent another ten seconds playing out different scenarios in my head. I realized the primary problem was not intubation; it was ventilation. If I could find a way to deliver oxygen to his lungs, I could buy enough time for another fiberoptic scope to arrive. Saturation was now at 40%. With only a few seconds left to make a decision, I chose to paralyze him without any sedation in order to save his life. Once he stopped moving, he became easier to ventilate. Now oxygen could be pushed into his lungs with only minor difficulty. His oxygen saturation started to rise—first to 50%, then 65%, then 70%. Eventually, it reached 90% as the second portable monitor arrived.

Then I inserted the fiberoptic scope into his mouth, guided it over his tongue, under his epiglottis, and into his trachea. He desaturated again. My heart rate stayed at 60. I slid the breathing tube over the scope into his trachea.

There were no complications.

§ THE SLOPE TO ENLIGHTENMENT §

As mentioned in the last chapter, too much early experience without the understanding of basic principles may result in false confidence. False confidence occurs when someone thinks they're an expert but is actually an amateur who doesn't realize how much they don't know. One might predict confidence would be proportional to ability—that is, experts exude the most confidence and amateurs exude the least. The reality is different. Rather than confidence increasing linearly with expertise, the most and least qualified people tend to display the most confidence. This unexpected pattern is called the Dunning-Kruger effect.[21]

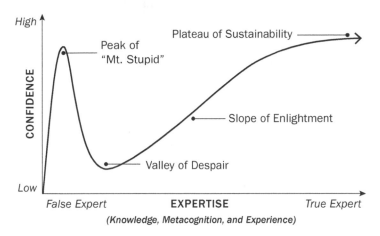

Figure 3-4

---

21 The Dunning-Kruger effect is named for cognitive psychologists David Dunning and Justin Kruger who observed those with objectively worse performance failed to evaluate themselves accurately. Their paper in the *Journal of Personal and Social Psychology* is titled "Unskilled and Unaware of It: How Difficulties in Recognizing One's Own Incompetence Lead to Inflated Self-Assessments."

Medical students and residents are treated sternly by their attendings to push them off Mount Stupid through the Valley of Despair. That's why residents seem so frustrated; the neural wiring of their brains and cognitive processes are rapidly evolving. Growth is inherently painful and frustrating. Young physicians must first learn how much they don't know so they can recognize the limits of their knowledge.

True experts are located at the second peak of the graph. False experts are represented by the first peak of the graph. Without the proper knowledge, metacognition, and experience, false experts cannot sort through uncertainty in a constructive manner. Without the nervous system to silence System 1, they tend to make shortsighted choices that cause additional second- and third-order consequences. In medicine, this equates to treating symptoms rather than addressing the cause of the underlying disease. Outside of the hospital, it equates to accepting limited short-term benefits at the expense of large future liabilities. Over time, these liabilities organize into Black Swans.

As our world becomes more complex, Systems 1 and 2 can be used to make better decisions. They were not described by physicians, but we utilize them because we want the best outcomes for our patients. We force each other to suffer through many years of frustrating training to make sure we become excellent decision makers. Now, at the end of my anesthesiology training, I finally feel comfortable managing medical complexity independently. More importantly, I can perform in complex domains, such as airway emergencies.

In this chapter, I've shared my long journey of becoming confident within complex systems. I learned to acknowledge reality for what it was rather than acting like it was a simple system. I invested the time and effort in order to gain the expertise needed to thrive in my new uncertain environment. I realized there are two ways to deal with ambiguity: the easy way and the correct way. The easy way is consistent with a simple system perspective and the correct way is consistent with a complex system perspective.

In the easy way, people avoid stress and ambiguity. They opt for the easiest, most efficient, most obvious way possible. The problem is that decisions in System 1 can lead to premature closure—deciding on an immediate, incorrect course of action rather than systematically working through uncertainty in a constructive manner. To thrive in complex environments, you must be able to tolerate uncomfortable periods of uncertainty in order to find the correct solution. Accepting limited short-term losses is often necessary to make the best decision.

In simple systems, learning is linear, predictable, and measurable. In complex systems, learning is often unclear, frustrating, and demoralizing. Objective reality doesn't care about your feelings or goals. Progress is irregular and not always seen, but that doesn't mean progress isn't happening. It's easy to feel defeated and give up to preserve your ego rather than learning to make real decisions.

Once I transitioned into System 2, my happiness increased exponentially because I didn't feel the need to avoid complexity or ambiguity. My relationships with nurses and other physicians improved. Patients seemed to like me more. But before I could transition, I had to hit rock bottom. I had to let go of my previous perception of how I thought the world *should* work and accept how it *actually* worked.

In our new world, synergy exists whether we think it does or not. Our outcomes will depend on whether we choose to accept its existence and how we choose to manage synergistic events. Whenever two simple systems interact, synergy is created. If that synergy is not accounted for in future decisions, it will continue to grow until it organizes into a Black Swan. The better option is to learn how to manage synergy so benefits can be harvested and catastrophes avoided. Although it can be tempting to treat the world as a simple system, denial will only lead to more Black Swans.

This concludes the first part of the book. In it, we defined synergy, Black Swans, complex systems, and simple systems. These concepts will be woven into the rest of the book. Now that we know how to characterize uncertainty, we can move on to applications of these concepts. In the next part of the book, we will dive into Black Swan management.

PART II

Managing Black Swans

CHAPTER 4

Monitors

"A turkey is fed for 1,000 days by a butcher, and every day confirms to the turkey and the turkey's economics department and the turkey's risk management department and the turkey's analytical department that the butcher loves turkeys, and every day brings more confidence to the statement. But on day 1,001 there will be a surprise for the turkey."

—Nassim Taleb

"Victorious warriors win first and then go to war, while defeated warriors go to war first and then seek to win."

—Sun Tzu, *The Art of War*

My patient was a 13-year-old girl with chronic right thigh pain intractable to medication and physical therapy. On this particular day, she was scheduled for a femoral neuroplasty to remove redundant soft tissue potentially causing inflammation around the right femoral nerve. We took her to the operating room, induced general anesthesia, then intubated her uneventfully. She was young and healthy. I always look forward to healthy patients. They are a welcome break from life-and-death emergencies.

About an hour into the case, I heard the ventilator alarm. Then the pulse oximeter tone changed. I looked at my monitors for three seconds, texted my attending to come immediately, then ran out of the room. I located an albuterol inhaler and returned to the room within 15 seconds. At that point, my patient's oxygen saturation was 80% and dropping. I unloaded ten puffs of the albuterol inhaler into her endotracheal tube. However, her oxygen saturation continued dropping.

It hovered at 70% without improvement. I gave her another ten puffs of albuterol. Finally, her oxygen saturation started climbing. She was safe…for now. By the time my attending arrived less than five minutes later, the situation was under control. Over the next 30 minutes, her oxygen saturation climbed to 85%. The surgeon and operating room nurse didn't notice anything had happened.

I had just treated my first bronchospasm. A bronchospasm is a sudden contraction of the upper airway smooth muscle that narrows bronchi to a dangerously small diameter. The narrow bronchi cannot exchange air, then oxygen cannot be exchanged in the lungs, and ultimately the patient's oxygen levels fall. If untreated, they will fall to dangerously low levels, eventually causing cardiac arrest. Thankfully, one important factor changed the outcome of this situation: I had monitors.

§ MEASURING SYNERGY §

Anesthesiology is 99% routine and 1% panic. Unfortunately, no one knows when the 1% panic will occur. Sometimes healthy patients have life-threatening complications and sometimes sick patients have no complications. The operating room does not have friends, only guests. And those guests never know when they are overstaying their welcome.

In the operating room, synergy covertly organizes until it becomes a Black Swan. The problem is, synergistic interactions often occur outside of our perspective. We only know they exist because complications exist. Even though synergy cannot be directly observed, it can be indirectly measured. By indirectly measuring specific simple systems in the operating room, anesthesiologists can predict possible synergistic interactions, then take early action to prevent Black Swans. This indirect measurement is the first step to managing Black Swans, and for us, it comes in the form of monitors.

Over the last 70 years, anesthesiologists incorporated monitors into clinical practice to detect harmful synergy before it organizes into a Black Swan. Our first and most important monitor is our brain. All other monitors are useless if we don't understand what those monitors mean. That's why anesthesiologists need the training of medical school and intern year—to understand how our monitors relate to the anatomical and physiological changes during surgery. These monitors measure blood pressure, heart rate, oxygen saturation, and temperature, among others.

The American Society of Anesthesiology (ASA) standard monitors are noninvasive blood pressure, continuous pulse oximetry, continuous electrocardiogram (cEKG), and temperature. These monitors represent the minimum level of synergy detection for safe anesthetics. Blood pressure must be measured at least every five minutes. It warns of Black Swans associated with low blood pressure such as anesthetic overdose, bleeding, and heart failure. Pulse oximetry measures the amount of oxygen in blood. It warns of Black Swans associated with hypoxia, such as bronchospasms. cEKG measures the electrical activity of the heart. It warns of Black Swans associated with cardiac function, such as cardiac arrythmias and heart attacks. Temperature monitoring warns of Black Swans associated with hypothermia. These monitors detect synergy so the anesthesiologist knows when Black Swans are likely to occur.[22]

Useful monitors have three characteristics:

1. **Early**. Monitors must grant enough time between synergy detection and a Black Swan for a meaningful change in management. Even seconds are enough.
2. **Qualitative**. Monitors measure a specific change in a simple system. Anesthesiologists are required to learn about the physics and chemistry behind their monitors, the anesthesia machine, and even the electromagnetic principles of surgical instruments. We need to know exactly what our monitors mean in order to interpret them correctly in the context of a complicated clinical situation. Every monitor has limitations, false positives, and false negatives.
3. **Quantitative**. Monitor measurement range must be proportional to the risk of a Black Swan. For example, pulse oximetry is most accurate between 70% and 90%. Coincidentally, this is the range where a change in clinical management is most likely to prevent life-threatening hypoxia. Anything less than 70% is an emergency regardless of the number. Anything more than 90% is generally not an emergency.

Other monitors include arterial blood pressure, central venous pressure, pulmonary arterial pressure, motor-evoked potentials, somatosensory-evoked potentials, transesophageal echocardiography, and cerebral oximetry. When an airway device is utilized, such as a breathing tube, capnography is recommended. Capnography measures the amount of carbon dioxide in exhaled breaths. It is an indirect measure of ventilation. For the purpose of this

---

22 More information about standard ASA monitors can be found at asahq.org/
standards-and-guidelines/standards-for-basic-anesthetic-monitoring.

chapter, we will focus on monitors used for my bronchospasm: pulse oximetry and capnography.

§ A BRIEF HISTORY OF PULSE OXIMETRY AND CAPNOGRAPHY §

Pulse oximetry is based on optical physics principles developed in the 1800s and early 1900s. Many high school students may recognize these principles as the Beer-Lambert law or Beer's law. In 1852, physicist August Beer discovered light shone through a substance dissolved in a solvent is absorbed in a predictable pattern. Then in 1860, German scientists used this pattern to develop analytical spectroscopy, the use of light to measure the chemical composition of solids, liquids, and gases. In the 1930s, Dr. Karl Matthes applied analytical spectroscopy to the different wavelengths of light reflected by hemoglobin in its oxygenated and deoxygenated states.

For the first time in history, the oxygen saturation of hemoglobin could be quantitatively measured, but the device had several practical limitations. Over the next 40 years, those practical limitations were solved by the US military and academic physiologists. Then in 1972, a young Japanese bioengineer named Takuo Aoyagi figured out how to use arterial pulsations to better calibrate the device. Modern pulse oximetry was born.

Although Aoyagi's employer, Nihon Kohden Corporation, did not see the potential in his innovation, others did. In 1979, Biox Technology was founded in Denver, Colorado, USA, and in 1981 Nellcor Company was formed in Hayward, California, USA. Nellcor employed anesthesiologist Dr. Mark Yelderman, who introduced the pulse oximetry device at the 1983 ASA annual conference. By 1986, the ASA adopted pulse oximetry as a standard monitor. Interestingly, there are no clinical trials showing pulse oximetry decreases mortality during surgery. Keep in mind there are also no clinical trials showing parachutes decrease death during skydiving. Despite the lack of data, I doubt you could find people willing to administer anesthesia without a pulse oximeter or skydive without a parachute.[23]

The first time I understood the importance of a pulse oximeter was during my fourth year of medical school on my pediatric anesthesiology rotation. I was with a third-year resident for the day. He extubated an adorable three-year-old girl after an uncomplicated hernia operation. After our attending anesthesiologist, the surgeon, and the nurse had left the room, the patient's oxygen saturation suddenly dropped to 60%.

The resident immediately gave me an oxygen mask connected to the anesthesia machine. He instructed me to hold the mask to the patient's face with both hands. He quickly turned a few dials on the anesthesia machine. I didn't dare look away from the child's face. I watched her lips turn blue in front of my eyes. I remember thinking, *I really hope this guy knows what he is doing.* After an intense 30 seconds, the child was breathing normally again. Her oxygen saturation improved immediately. She woke up ten minutes later without further complications.

The resident had expertly managed a laryngospasm, a complication most commonly seen in pediatric patients when the vocal cords spontaneously close without warning. Without the pulse oximeter, we might not have recognized the complication in time to treat it appropriately. Our first sign of a problem would have been the child turning blue, and that sign might have come too late. If it had happened in the hallway on the way to the recovery room, we would not have had the proper equipment to treat it.

---

23   A succinct 2017 review article is "Beat to Beat: A Measured Look at the History of Pulse Oximetry" by Dr. Antoinette Van Meter, et al.

Capnography, which measures $EtCO_2$ (pronounced "end-tidal carbon dioxide"), is the other monitor that changed the landscape of anesthesiology. The measurement of CO_2 from human breath was first reported by Irish physicist John Tyndall in 1865. Then in 1928, American physicist John Aitken and English physician Dr. Archibald Clark-Kennedy made multiple practical advances that led to the first volumetric capnogram. After wartime applications, the technology entered clinical medicine in 1955 when the first capnographic profiles of human respiration were recorded in the anesthesiology literature. By the 1970s, $EtCO_2$ changes were linked to clinical changes in patients.

In 1978, clinical capnography was introduced in the United States at the World Congress of Critical Care Medicine. Initially, it was thought to be "of little value." Then a Canadian malpractice insurer granted premium discounts to anesthesiologists who used capnography during their cases because it decreased esophageal intubation claims. Esophageal intubation is placing the breathing tube into the esophagus instead of the trachea. If unrecognized, the patient will die from hypoxia. The technology became widespread in the 1990s. It eliminated mortality associated with esophageal intubation and greatly improved the safety of sedation especially in endoscopy procedures like colonoscopies.[24]

I'm grateful for this technology. I have accidentally intubated the esophagus twice in my life...so far. Both times, I immediately recognized my mistake, then reintubated safely. Both cases proceeded without further complications or patient harm. In my bronchospasm case, I recognized the capnography waveform

---

24 Michael Jaffe gave a review of capnography history in his 2011 ASA conference presentation titled "Volumetric Capnography—A Brief History." A more comprehensive history was published in 2004. Its title is *Capnography: Clinical Aspects*, edited by J. S. Gravenstein, Michael Jaffe, and David Palus.

changed in a way consistent with a bronchospasm. Looking back, I bet the resident who recognized the laryngospasm confirmed his suspicion with capnography, just as I did with the bronchospasm.

§ SITTING IN THE WOODS §

Although technology can help us prevent Black Swans, we must never underestimate our five senses. As a resident, I had the privilege of training with Dr. Anahat Dhillon. Her kind demeanor betrays her depth of expertise and high expectations for herself and her trainees. When something is good, she will tell you. When something is not good, she will also tell you. Your fate is your choice. She is simply the messenger.

One day, I was working with her during a robotic pancreatic resection (coincidentally, Dr. Nissen was the surgeon). At one point, Dr. Dhillon asked me to close my eyes, then guess the heart rate and oxygen saturation. The beep-beep-beep sound in the operating room is made up of two components: the rate of the beeping is set by the heart rate of the EKG, and the pitch of the sound is determined by the percent oxygen saturation of the pulse oximeter. High-pitch tones mean a higher saturation (>90%) and low-pitch sounds mean a lower saturation (<90%). Because the tone of the beep changes based on the oxygen saturation, an anesthesiologist can know both values just by listening.

After about 30 minutes of practice, I could be within five beats per minute of the true value for the heart rate and within 2% of the oxygen saturation. Since that day with Dr. Dhillon, I remember that my ears independently give me information about the entire operating room. I learned to listen to the surgeon's voice, the electrocautery, the suction, and the circulating nurse to understand all activity around me.

This practice is like meditating in the middle of a forest. At first, you will hear nothing. Eventually, you will become acutely aware of all activity around you: the sounds of the leaves rustling, animals walking, water running, and birds calling. I played a game with myself where I would close my eyes and guess what was happening in the operating room, and then I'd look around to see if I was correct. Over time, I could tell what the surgeons were doing just by the tone of their voices and the instruments they asked for.

A year after my case with Dr. Dhillon, while on call, I anesthetized a patient receiving a liver transplant. The time was about 2:00 a.m. I had worked all day and then started the transplant early in the evening. Initially, the case went well. The failing liver was removed, a new liver was inserted in its place, and then the hepatic artery and portal vein were anastomosed to the patient's native vasculature. Before working on the common bile duct, the surgeons repaired an incision in the patient's groin.

Then I noticed the suction catheters near the liver were making a characteristic sound. I asked the surgeons to reexplore the liver bed for an arterial bleed. At first they resisted, but because I persisted, they finally humored my request. As they lifted the liver, multiple bright red jets of arterial blood appeared. My junior resident demanded I tell her how I knew about the arterial bleed.

I smiled, then said, "Close your eyes and tell me what the heart rate is."

Monitors are not designed to look at routine events. They are meant to identify signs of large, uncommon events. I have only seen one bronchospasm over my eight years of medical training, but I recognized it immediately and treated it without hesitation. Ninety-nine percent of the time, monitors are retrospectively not necessary, but that doesn't mean we shouldn't use them. There is no way to measure the number of complications *avoided* because of monitors.

In anesthesiology, Black Swans are unavoidable. The patient, anesthesia drugs, and surgery produce incredible amount of synergy. The synergy organizes into single events that have a disproportionally large effect on human physiology, sometimes large enough to cause death within minutes. Examples include bronchospasm, laryngospasm, or arterial bleed after liver transplant.

One percent is a lot, especially in anesthesiology. For perspective, an anesthesiologist with a 1% mortality rate is no different than a highly motivated serial killer; he or she would kill about one patient every month (assuming 100 cases per month). His or her medical license would be gone in less than a year. A 0.1% mortality rate is one patient death every ten months. Still in serial killer territory. A 0.01% mortality rate is one patient death every ten years. Now you are just negligent. A 0.001% mortality rate is one death every 100 years. Still too dangerous. In 2018, the mortality rate was 0.00051%. One death every 179 years.

§ SYNERGISTIC WEALTH §

Monitors are most useful in large, complex systems that produce excessive amounts of synergy because those are the systems in which Black Swans are most likely to occur. In anesthesiology, high synergy means multiple medical problems, emergency surgery, rare diseases, old age, and taking multiple medications. It also means more complicated surgeries, such as organ transplantation, heart surgery involving cardiopulmonary bypass, major vascular surgery, and spine surgery.

The operating room is not the only highly synergistic system where monitors are useful. Other synergistic arenas include economics, finance, and banking. With the significant deregulation in the last 50 years, the US economy has become increasingly synergistic. Deregulation is not a bad thing per se; it has exponentially increased the wealth of the United States by encouraging new ideas and innovations. The United States is still the richest country in the world by a large margin. From the outside, we look remarkably successful. So why is our society imploding?

We used to live in a pure gaussian world, where wealth was tied to physical quantities, such as land, people, and factories. Synergistic quantities, such as stocks, corporations, and legal entities, introduced a new kind of wealth based on the *interactions between gaussian parts* rather than the *actions of an individual.*

Below is a chart of gaussian and synergistic wealth. This is analogous to the chart of the gaussian and synergistic worlds.

	GAUSSIAN WEALTH	SYNERGISTIC WEALTH
CHARACTERISTICS	Finite quantities bound by physical laws	Infinite quantities without physical bounds
	Exists in objective reality	Exists in subjective reality
EXAMPLES	Paper money (as long as the federal government exists)	Stocks
	Gold	Corporations
	Silver	Bonds
	People	Legal entities
	Factories	Art
	Time	Intellectual property

Figure 4-1

Synergistic quantities can grow without bounds, whereas gaussian quantities are limited by the physical world. Mathematically speaking, synergistic wealth grows exponentially while gaussian wealth grows linearly. Below is a chart showing the difference between linear and exponential growth over time. The X-axis is time and the Y-axis is total value.[25]

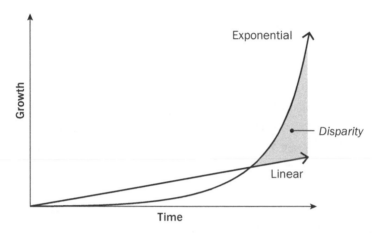

Figure 4-2

Over time, synergistic quantities become much larger than the gaussian quantities. This becomes a problem when extreme amounts of synergistic wealth cause structural asymmetries.

A structural asymmetry is a single point of data much, much larger than the average. Generally, a structural asymmetry is more than a hundred times larger or smaller than the most common event in a distribution. In statistics, distributions with structural asymmetries are said to have skew. Positive skew means the asymmetry is

25   Think of gaussian wealth as a savings account and synergistic wealth as a stock portfolio. If you deposited $100 every month for 20 years, the savings account would contain about $24,000. That same money invested into a stock portfolio with a 5% annual return rate would yield $40,000 over the same 20 years: a $16,000 difference. If the time period was 40 years, the difference would increase to about $100,000 ($48,000 vs. $145,000).

caused by very large outliers. Negative skew means the asymmetry is caused by very small outliers. A structural asymmetry occurs when a system contains an outlier so large or small that it makes the mode diverge from the median and mean.[26]

Below is a diagram showing how large outliers cause skew in gaussian distributions:

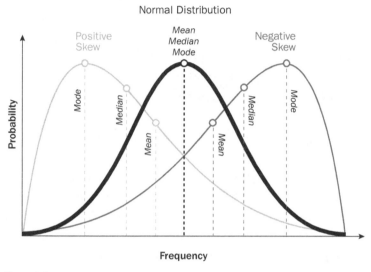

Figure 4-3

Does this look familiar? Perhaps like the synergistic and gaussian distributions from Chapter 1?

The larger the outlier, the greater effect it has on its system. For example, if 50% of the world's grapes came from the same vineyard, the supply (and cost) of grapes could drastically change

26 Mean, median, and mode are different ways to describe an average. Mean is all of the numbers added together divided by the total number of numbers. Median is the middle number if all of them were arranged from low to high. Mode is the most common number. The differences between them are useful because they describe how much a skewed distribution diverges from a normal distribution. The more skew, the more the three averages diverge.

based on a single unexpected storm. If that 50% was instead supplied by 50 smaller vineyards in different places, each growing 1% of the total, bad weather for a single vineyard would affect only 1% of the total supply. Bad weather for the large 50% vineyard would be a Black Swan for winemakers. Bad weather for one of the smaller 1% vineyards would be a minor inconvenience.

Observable, tangible quantities fall into gaussian distributions. Things like height, weight, and blood pressure are all accurately described by the normal distribution because they are tied to physical laws. In these systems, no structural asymmetries can exist. You can't have a person who is 1,000 feet tall or a blood pressure of 8,000/2,000 (normal is 120/80 mmHg). However, synergistic quantities don't have to follow gaussian laws. That means we need an entirely new way to describe and monitor them.

As synergistic quantities grow without bounds, they cause greater and greater skew from the normal distribution (pure gaussian world). The mode, median, and mean diverge because a small number of outliers warp the normal distribution. Those large outliers tend to produce Black Swans because they have a disproportionately large impact on the system compared to the average component.

Below are skewed distributions with both large and small structural asymmetries:

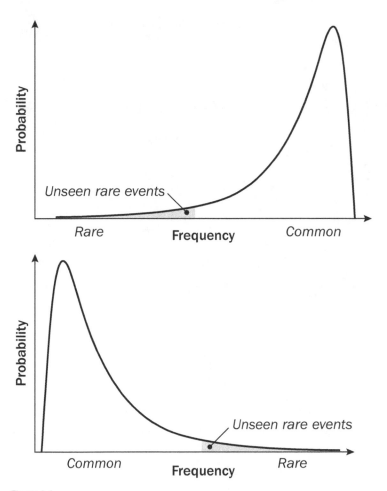

Figure 4-4

The positive skew pattern is observable in the United States' income distribution, pictured below.

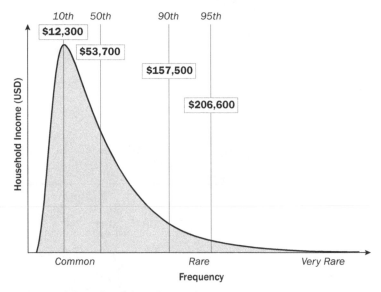

Distribution of Household Income 2014

Source: U.S. Census Bureau, Current Population Survey, 2015 Annual Social and Economic Supplement.

Figure 4-5

The reason the distribution is skewed is because the United States has a few people who have synergistic income more than 10,000x larger than the mode ($12,300). For perspective, the difference between the 50th and 95th percentile is only a factor of four.

The large outliers located on the far right side of the distribution are so much bigger than the mode that if the data was normally distributed and the distance between the 50th and 95th percentile was one inch, the distance from the 50th percentile to a million dollars of income would be six inches to the right. For perspective, $10 million would be 65 inches (5.3 feet, height of an average woman), $100 million would be 653 inches (54 feet), and $1 billion would be 6,540 inches (545 feet, 1.5 American football fields). Those are impressive asymmetries!

Theoretically, deregulation is supposed to decrease these asymmetries by allowing everyone to participate equally. If there are low barriers to entry and minimal regulation, it would theoretically be difficult for one entity to become a structural asymmetry. This works...up to a point. Eventually, if a legal entity becomes large enough, it can use its size to rewrite laws in order to grow larger. Now the legal entity is no longer playing by gaussian rules and therefore is not affected by gaussian laws. This is why large economic institutions like billionaires, international corporations, and governments introduce structural asymmetries into our lives.

Synergistic growth eventually leads to structural asymmetries and Black Swans. Structural asymmetries in anesthesiology are large changes in human physiology, such as massive bleeding, very low or high heart rate, very low or very high blood pressure, or low oxygen saturation. This is why anesthesiologists designed monitors to locate them before they cause irreversible damage.

In the operating room, irreversible damage equals death. In the world of finance, irreversible damage equals a financial disaster like the stock market crash of 1929, the Great Recession of the early 2000s, or the subprime mortgage housing crisis of 2008. In finance, bailouts exist. In anesthesiology, they do not. Your patient just dies.

Finance, entrepreneurship, and corporations are not inherently bad things. I would argue they are the engines of economic prosperity. However, an entity that protects its wealth at the expense of the system it serves can ultimately suppress healthy competition and create Black Swans. Monitors might be a good way to measure these highly synergistic systems for signs of Black Swans.

§ MONITORS FOR THE 21ST CENTURY §

We can learn from anesthesiologists and develop monitors to detect unstable synergy before it can organize into the catastrophic Black Swans. Our world is likely to be increasingly synergistic in the future. That is not inherently a bad thing, but it does require a different way to think about risk. The risks associated with gaussian quantities are inherently different from risks associated with synergistic quantities.

Gaussian systems thrive by creating rules based off the average. In a normal curve, the mean, median, and mode are the same value, so the term *average* is specific enough. In complex systems, the mean, median, and mode are all different—sometimes very different. Our perception of a complex system will be warped if we assume the three averages are the same. In a highly skewed distribution, the mean and median can be a factor of 100 (or more) larger than the mode. Synergistic systems are fundamentally different from gaussian ones and therefore require different rules for their management.

Synergistic systems thrive by making rules based off outliers. Twenty-first-century monitors should focus on structural asymmetries rather than the mode. Disproportionately large synergistic entities such as multinational corporations, billionaires, and governments introduce structural asymmetries because of their size. If they are not highly regulated, they will produce destructive Black Swans in order to feed their unlimited growth. In our modern world, legal entities sometimes exist for too long and become too big for their own good.

They eventually dominate, suppress, and then destroy the gaussian systems that created them. When those synergistic entities become too big *and* prioritize their survival at the expense of the system, they become a dangerous liability instead of a symbol of free enterprise. People who rely on gaussian wealth for their livelihood will be economically and politically dominated by those who have synergistic wealth. As the old saying goes, "You either die a hero or live long enough to become the villain."

Twenty-first-century monitors should focus on outliers, synergy, and Black Swans. By defining, studying, and measuring these quantities in systematic ways, we might be able to harvest the benefits of synergy while avoiding catastrophes. To do this, we must shift our mindset from the gaussian to the synergistic. Pure gaussian quantities will regulate themselves over time because they can only grow to a maximum size and are subject to immediate feedback from the rest of the system.

Synergistic factors require additional monitoring because they can grow to an infinite size without regard to the rest of the system. For this reason, anesthesia monitors focus on the things that destroy the complex system of the human body rather than common events. We must intervene during the rare events, figure out why they happened, and then correct the problem before the Black Swan kills our patient.

Ninety-nine percent of the time, synergy cannot organize into a complication because anesthesiologists make small gradual changes to minimize the chance of a large asymmetry. However, 1% of the time, we have to intervene quickly to treat a Black Swan. In the next chapter, we will discuss how to approach the 1% of times where intervention is necessary.

CHAPTER 5

The Time Horizon

"The formulation of the problem is often more essential than its solution, which may be merely a matter of mathematical or experimental skill."

—ALBERT EINSTEIN

"It is a capital mistake to theorize before one has data. Insensibly one begins to twist facts to suit theories, instead of theories to suit facts."

—SHERLOCK HOLMES, *A SCANDAL IN BOHEMIA*

As an organism grows, its cells copy their genetic material and then divide. Theoretically, the daughter cells should be the same as their parent cells, but sometimes mistakes occur. If enough harmful mutations (mistakes) develop in a single cell, then the cell can divide uncontrollably. Uncontrolled cell division is called a tumor. If the tumor invades additional parts of the body, it is called cancer. Cancer is a Black Swan of cell division.

Oftentimes, neoplasia and dysplasia, two intermediate states between normal cells and cancer, are monitored and then treated before cancer develops. Cancer screening tests, such as colonoscopies, mammograms, and PAP smears are examples of synergy monitors. The harmful synergy from cell division can be extinguished if it is caught early.

"Curing cancer" is different from curing a simple disease, such as a bacterial infection. Simple diseases, like infections, arise from an unnecessary external process. Synergistic diseases like cancer arise from essential processes like cell division.

Cancer cannot be cured because cell division is required for growth, repair of damaged cells, and maintaining the body's vital functions. It can be treated such that it inflicts minimal harm, especially so it doesn't kill us, but the essential process producing cancer cannot be stopped. The vast majority of the time cell division occurs without problems, but eventually it can become cancer. Like cancer treatment, this chapter will address what to do when a Black Swan occurs (that 1% of the time).

The management can be divided into three strategies depending on the level of uncertainty present. The strategies focus on what you don't know rather than what you do know. They are decisive action, *via negativa*, and buying time. All three change the time horizon of the Black Swan. First, we will define what a time horizon is, then talk about how it is applied.

A time horizon is a fixed point in the future when an event will occur. In the case of cancer, that something is death. If doctors increase the time horizon of death beyond the life span of their patient, the cancer is functionally neutralized. Similarly, the goal of anesthesiologists is to increase the time horizon of patient death beyond the time horizon of their anesthetic. If we can put death into remission during surgery, then our patient will wake up unharmed.

Below is a chart explaining how time horizons work. The top patient has untreated cancer. She gets cancer when she is young, is untreated, and dies prematurely because the time horizon of death from cancer is shorter than the time horizon of death from old age. The bottom patient has treated cancer. The treatment extends the time horizon of death from cancer beyond her natural life span. She still technically has cancer, but it no longer has a meaningful effect on her life span. She is in permanent remission.

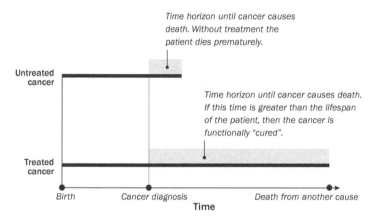

Figure 5-1

The same concept is used by anesthesiologists to control the time horizon of patient death due to a Black Swan event. Effective time horizon management is based on how much we know and don't know about the problem. We either act quickly before the Black Swan can kill our patient, or we delay the lethal effects of the Black Swan long enough to figure out the source of the underlying synergy.

First, let's consider Black Swan time horizon management when the problem and solution are both known with a high level of certainty.

§ DECISIVE ACTION §

After a full day of cases, I met Dr. Avi Gereboff in operating room 8-1. His easygoing demeanor underestimates his knowledge and experience. The anesthesiology residents, including myself, usually meet him on call during liver transplants. We spend the night learning about pulmonary artery catheters, hemodynamics, blood coagulation, and liver transplant anatomy. I have anesthetized several liver transplants in residency—one I remember in particular.

The first part of the operation was uneventful. The failing liver was removed, and the new one was placed inside of the patient. Then the new liver was connected to the patient's venous system via suturing of the hepatic portal vein (3), infrahepatic inferior vena cava (2), and suprahepatic inferior vena cava (1).[27]

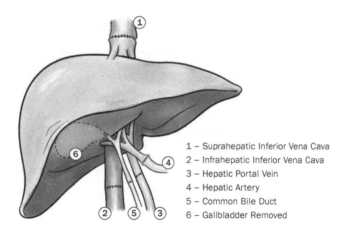

1 – Suprahepatic Inferior Vena Cava
2 – Infrahepatic Inferior Vena Cava
3 – Hepatic Portal Vein
4 – Hepatic Artery
5 – Common Bile Duct
6 – Gallbladder Removed

Figure 5-2

---

27 Transplanted livers usually have their associated gallbladders removed. I will leave a comprehensive discussion of liver transplant surgical anatomy to my hepatobiliary surgical colleagues.

After the veins were connected, everyone in the room became silent. The patient's blood pressure suddenly dropped from 140/90 to 60/20 mmHg. The inferior vena cava suture line (2) ruptured. All venous blood from the lower half of the body was spilling into the abdomen, approximately 1–2 L/min. Dr. Gereboff recognized the complication in less than a second. He knew he could not keep up with this blood loss, so he immediately turned up our transfusion system to its maximum transfusion capacity of 500 cc/minute and turned off all anesthetics as he directed me to draw up multiple presser medications to increase the heart rate and vascular tone. I also cleared off the patient's chest in case we needed to start chest compressions.

I am thankful to work with excellent surgeons and anesthesiologists who are more than able to handle complications. In this case, the hepatobiliary surgery fellow expertly controlled the bleeding and then repaired the large blood vessel. The patient's blood pressure steadily rose back to normal levels. The case proceeded without further complications.

The key to addressing this Black Swan was keeping the patient alive long enough for the surgeons to control the bleeding. Quick, decisive action is necessary in situations where the problem and the solution are known with high certainty. Both lie in the first layer of knowledge.

§ *VIA NEGATIVA* §

What do we do when the problem lies in the first layer of knowledge, but the solution lies in the second or third layer? How do we approach Black Swans when we know the problem but don't know the solution?

The best way to deal with these problems is to systemically eliminate cognitive blindness to increase the chance of finding the correct solution. Anesthesiologists use a technique called *via negativa*. One notable case occurred during my third year of residency when I was called to anesthetize a patient for emergency spine surgery.[28]

My patient was a 46-year-old man originally transferred for cardiac bypass surgery, but he developed an infection next to his spinal cord resulting in bilateral leg weakness. This specific infection, called an epidural abscess, is a surgical emergency because the infection can quickly damage the spinal cord or spread to the brain.

My attending, Dr. Brian Mendelson, and I took him to the operating room, intubated him, placed arterial and venous monitors, and then flipped him prone. Spine surgeries usually require the patient to be positioned prone (facedown) so the surgeon can access the spine through the back. After we flipped him, we could no longer ventilate him. For an anesthesiologist, being unable to ventilate a patient with an endotracheal tube is a nightmare. This meant we had about two minutes to flip him back over, or he would die of hypoxia. It didn't help that he weighed more than 300 pounds (>138 kg). His lips turned blue just as we flipped him back into supine position.

We had no idea why we could not ventilate him. He had no significant pulmonary disease before surgery. Neither of us had

---

28   *Via negativa*, also called apophatic theology, attempts to approach God by speaking in terms of what He is not. This form of theological thinking inherently implies the understanding of the subject (God) is beyond the scope of human knowledge. Although this book is about anesthesiology, I still think this form of thinking is useful for describing problems we cannot fully understand. Nassim Taleb writes extensively about it in his book *Antifragile: Things that Gain from Disorder*.

seen this scenario before. Over the next 30 minutes, we addressed every reversible cause we could think of. *Via negativa* gets you closer to the truth by eliminating untrue possibilities. If you can eliminate enough possibilities, whatever remains must be the truth, assuming the truth is knowable.

We then tried to prone him again but with similar results. Dr. Mendelson suspected his lungs were filled with fluid from untreated heart failure. He probably needed further treatment before returning to the operating room. Usually, patients with pulmonary edema due to heart failure require extra oxygen, have abnormal vital signs, and cannot breathe normally. They have obvious clinical signs such as coughing, poor oxygenation, and leg swelling. Our patient had none of these.

This patient's physiology seemed to be fine, but it clearly wasn't. Despite the risk of permanent lower extremity paralysis, Dr. Mendelson recommended postponing the case, admitting the patient to the cardiac surgical ICU (CSICU), then obtaining cardiology and pulmonology consultations. We predicted he would need several days of diuresis so the excess fluid could be cleared from his lungs. In the meantime, we hoped antibiotics would prevent the epidural abscess from enlarging.

The neurosurgeon begrudgingly accepted. We all understood the emergent nature of the surgery, but we also knew without ventilation, he would die within minutes. After four days of diuresis (giving medications to artificially increase urine output), he lost 8 kg (17 lb) of fluid weight.

He returned to the operating room, and the surgery proceeded without complications. Luckily for him, his epidural abscess did not enlarge while he was in the CSICU. He was eventually discharged to a nursing facility without neurological deficits. Months later, he returned for his cardiac bypass operation.

Our *via negativa* thinking narrowed the possibilities from common to uncommon, likely to unlikely. We correctly predicted his cardiac problem by eliminating all other possibilities. As Sherlock Holmes would say, "When you have eliminated the impossible, whatever remains, however improbable, must be the truth."[29]

§ BUYING TIME §

The third type of time horizon management occurs when both the cause and solution are unknown. These types of problems are notoriously difficult to solve. In addition to figuring out the cause behind the disease process, anesthesiologists must also treat the symptoms of the disease so our patients can survive until a permanent solution is found. An excellent example of this was how Dr. Bjørn Ibsen treated bulbar polio while a polio vaccine was being developed.

Dr. Bjørn Ibsen, a Danish anesthesiologist, had a problem. In the early 1900s, polio evolved into large epidemics in Europe and North America. During the 1940s and 1950s, the disease afflicted hundreds of thousands of people every year. Lockdowns, similar to the COVID-19 lockdowns in 2020, frequently occurred to stop the spread of the virus. The modern polio vaccine did not exist yet. In early 1952, Copenhagen prepared for an unusually

---

29   The full line is from *The Sign of the Four*: "How often have I said to you that when you have eliminated the impossible, whatever remains, *however improbable*, must be the truth? We know that he did not come through the door, the window, or the chimney. We also know that he could not have been concealed in the room, as there is no concealment possible. When, then, did he come?" Here, Holmes is trying to explain his thinking to Watson. Note Holmes first excludes the impossible (possibilities he knows he doesn't know, third layer of knowledge) prior to using deduction.

large polio epidemic. The problem was, they didn't have enough staff, money, or equipment. They were desperate for a solution.

Polio is a neurological disease. Its scientific name, *poliomyelitis*, is a combination of the Greek words *polio* meaning "gray," *myelo* referring to the inside of the spinal cord, and *–itis* meaning "inflammation." The virus causes inflammation of gray neurons located in the anterior (front half) of the spinal cord.

It is transmitted via fecal-oral route. It replicates in the gastrointestinal (GI) tract of its human host, then spreads to its next victim when the host touches other people or objects without proper hand hygiene. When inside its new host, it replicates in the GI tract. Then it moves to the spinal cord where it causes inflammation of motor neurons responsible for voluntary movement of the extremities.

In severe cases, the virus can move up the spinal cord into the brainstem, called bulbar polio. Bulbar refers to the cerebellum, pons, and medulla—the structures at the base of the brain. The virus disables the nerves responsible for moving the diaphragm, and the victim suffocates. Paralysis usually improves over the course of two weeks; however, victims may have residual paralysis of their lower extremities after the disease passes.

Since 1928, a rudimentary ventilator, the iron lung, was used to help bulbar polio patients breathe until their paralysis improved. Unfortunately for Dr. Ibsen, the iron lung had several practical limitations: it was expensive, difficult to maintain, required a dedicated experienced operator, and patients' secretions were difficult to manage; they sometimes traveled into the lungs causing a severe chemical pneumonia. Furthermore there was only one iron lung in the whole city of Copenhagen. In the first three weeks of the epidemic, 27 of 31 patients with bulbar polio died, an 87% mortality rate. Half of them were children.

Luckily, Dr. Ibsen had a plan. First, polio patients who developed the severe bulbar form would be given tracheostomies. *Stoma* is the Greek word for "hole." Therefore, a tracheostomy is a hole in the trachea. Through the hole, an endotracheal tube (*endo* means "inside") would be inserted. The tube was connected to a bag mask valve, a rubber bag that could be squeezed to force air through the endotracheal tube into the patient's lungs.

Ventilation could be achieved with easy management of secretions, reducing the incidence of aspiration pneumonia to zero. The bulbar polio patients were organized into a new ward where medical students squeezed the rubber bags for 24 hours a day in six- to eight-hour shifts under supervision of doctors and nurses. At the height of the epidemic, the ward had 105 beds.

Due to Dr. Ibsen's innovative polio treatment, the mortality rate decreased from about 90% to 25%. He even utilized recent advances in respiratory physiology to measure blood pH (measure of acid-base balance) to optimize the amount of ventilation. His use of positive pressure ventilation, organization of patients based on severity of disease, and efficient distribution of labor are considered the world's first ICU. Dr. Ibsen was the world's first intensive care physician.

Dr. Ibsen found a way to prevent patient death without curing the disease. His solution was to extend the time horizon of respiratory failure (death from polio) beyond that of the natural course of the disease. He didn't need to cure the disease; he only needed to extend the time horizon of its most dangerous manifestation.

Below is a summary of Black Swan time horizon management.

TYPE OF PROBLEM	MANAGEMENT
Certain problem, certain solution	Act quickly before Black Swan occurs
Certain problem, uncertain solution	Eliminate perceptive perception (*via negativa*)
Uncertain problem, uncertain solution	Delay time horizon of Black Swan to define the problem

Figure 5-3

§ POLIO AND COVID-19 §

President Franklin Delano Roosevelt was afflicted by a paralytic illness at age 39, presumed to be polio, rendering him paraplegic. In 1938, he founded the National Foundation for Infantile Paralysis to raise money for polio treatment and research. Today, it is known as the March of Dimes, and it spends most of its time improving the health of infants and their mothers.

In January 1938, the name March of Dimes was coined by Eddie Cantor, an American entertainer. He popularized a fundraising campaign where anyone could buy a pin for a dime the week before FDR's 56th birthday. Within a week, the White House received 40,000–50,000 letters and about $85,000 in dimes (the equivalent of about $1.5 million in 2020 dollars). Over the next 20 years, the foundation spent $233 million on polio patient care. More than 80% of American polio patients received medical care because of the foundation alone. Because of FDR's leadership in polio treatment and research, in 1946, the United States Mint placed his face on the dime, a design still used today. Go find a dime. See for yourself![30]

---

30 A brief history of the March of Dimes can be found in *Polio: An American Story* by David Ochinsky, pp. 43–79. More information about the Roosevelt dime can be found on the United States Mint website.

Finally in 1952, Dr. Jonas Salk and his team at the University of Pittsburgh invented the inactivated polio vaccine. By 1961, after nine years of vaccination campaigns, only 161 cases were reported in the United States. Sixty-seven years passed between the first polio outbreaks and the creation of an effective vaccine.[31]

The 1938 political and cultural responses to polio differ from the 2020 response to COVID-19. Citizens and some politicians downplayed the severity of the virus, refused to wear masks, and would not socially distance. Some people in the United States refuse to acknowledge the existence of the virus, instead labeling it an elaborate hoax. Why?

The differences between the two responses might be explained in terms of synergy. Polio spreads in a gaussian manner, and COVID-19 spreads in a synergistic manner.

Polio spreads via direct physical contact between people. Perceivable, measurable interventions decrease its spread in a predictable linear manner. Polio is highly symptomatic, which means infected people can be quickly identified and then quarantined. Unlike COVID-19, polio spread and prevention is gaussian.

COVID-19 spreads through the air in a synergistic manner, which is much harder to quantify or measure. COVID-19 is usually asymptomatic or mildly symptomatic. Symptoms usually develop after the disease is present instead of at the time of infection. COVID-19 challenges the gaussian idea that disease is limited to what we perceive—that is, symptoms equate to disease. In the synergistic world of COVID-19, symptoms and spread of disease

---

31 A succinct history of polio and its vaccines can be found at historyofvaccines.org/timeline/polio. A perspective of the mass vaccination campaign was published in 1984 by Dr. Albert Hinman. The title of his article is "Landmark Perspective: Mass Vaccination against Polio."

have little to do with each other. Cause and effect functionally do not exist.

The true burden of synergistic diseases like COVID-19 is much greater than the sum of symptomatic individuals. SARS-CoV-2 exhibits exponential growth in a population because it is difficult to detect. At first, the number of infected people increases slowly, and the disease seems like it's "not a big deal." Eventually, the disease infects more and more people at an uncontrollable rate. Hospitals fill up, then people die in record numbers. Like a sudden complication in the operating room, everything seems normal until a state of emergency occurs.

How do you explain these strange findings to someone who doesn't believe in synergy? From a gaussian perspective, COVID-19 is literally magic. The denial of COVID-19 is not illogical; it simply reflects a denial of synergy.

The acknowledgment of uncertainty and Black Swans is the first step to solving synergistic problems. In the gaussian world, the focus is on what we know. In the synergistic world, the focus is on what we don't know.

Again, we can learn from anesthesiologists, who assume the solution is outside their perspective and then work backward from uncertainty to certainty. This style of problem solving is called inductive reasoning, where evidence is synthesized into a general truth. Inductive reasoning is best suited to complex systems because it leaves room for synergistic events ($1 + 1 = 3$).

Deductive reasoning runs in the opposite direction. General rules are applied to evidence to determine what happened. This kind of reasoning works best in simple systems because it assumes all the rules are known. In complex systems, we cannot know all of the "rules," so relying solely on deductive reasoning will miss synergistic factors outside of our perspective. Applying deductive reasoning to synergistic problems like COVID-19 will underestimate their severity.[32]

We can use the same strategy to help make sense of the increasing uncertainty that defines our lives in the 21st century. If we want an interconnected world, we must be prepared to characterize, study, and manage its synergy.

As the world struggles to manage COVID-19, we must consider another important Black Swan management issue: how to divide resources during Black Swan events. With limited resources and time, what should be prioritized first? In order to answer that question, let's see what anesthesiologists do when their patients' hearts suddenly stop. The truth is both different and more interesting than what you see on television shows like *ER* and *Grey's Anatomy*.

---

32 Deduction and induction have relative strengths and weaknesses depending on the amount of uncertainty present. Induction is more useful when solving a unique problem; deduction is most useful when solving different iterations of a known pattern. Deduction takes away until reality matches theory; induction adds until theory matches reality.

CHAPTER 6

Code Blue

"Distributive justice isn't taking from a risk taker who earned his fortune honorably, it is keeping his probability of losing back his fortune very high."

—NASSIM TALEB

"Over the long term, symbiosis is more useful than parasitism."

—LARRY WALL, AMERICAN COMPUTER PROGRAMMER

After cardiac surgery, patients are admitted to the cardiac ICU. Most of the time, nothing happens. The patient arrives, the breathing tube is removed the first day, infusions of inotrope and presser medications are weaned down the second day, and chest tubes are removed the third day. Patients recover uneventfully over three to five days, and then they are transferred to a lower acuity hospital room.

Post-operative recovery usually goes according to plan…until it doesn't. They are at very high risk of developing sudden, life-threatening complications. Sometimes, the heart's electrical conduction system fails, the kidneys fail, or patients are taken back to the operating room for surgical exploration.

Sometimes patients can't make it to the operating room safely. In those situations, the chest is reopened in the ICU. All cardiac ICU rooms can transform into a cardiac operating room within minutes. Complications of the heart and lungs warrant the fastest interventions in medicine because the rest of the body relies on oxygenated blood to survive.

Oxygenated blood to the body is like electricity to New York City—without it, the entire system would fail within minutes. This is not true for all components of complex systems. For example, the body can live without a gallbladder, a colon, or an arm. New York City doesn't need 350 Starbucks or more than 3,000 coffee shops—they are a convenience rather than a necessity.[33]

In the complex system of the human body, the most essential organs are the brain, heart, and lungs. The brain is most essential of these three because it creates our identity. Then come the heart and lungs. After these three, the next most essential organs are the kidneys and liver. Then the organs that are beneficial but not technically essential include the stomach, intestines, and spleen. Their removal usually causes problems. Last, organs like the appendix and gallbladder are potentially helpful but do not serve an essential function.

This chapter will articulate what parts of a complex system should be prioritized during emergency situations. When medical Black Swans occur, such as a heart attack or pulmonary embolism (blood clot in lungs), patient lives are saved by correct triage of problems according to the essentialness of the organ system. Strategies perfected by physicians can be applied to other complex systems outside of the hospital.

---

33 A brief history of Starbucks Coffee in New York City can be found on the Starbucks website: stories.starbucks.com/stories/2018/a-brief-history-of-starbucks-in-new-york/.

§ HANDS OF GOD §

My second clinical rotation of medical school was the medical intensive care unit. One day, I arrived promptly at 6:45 a.m. to help the residents compile vital signs, urine output, and labs from the previous 24 hours. At 7:05 a.m., the overhead paging system announced, "Code Blue Karmanos Cancer Center fourth floor, Code Blue Karmanos Cancer Center fourth floor, Code Blue Karmanos Cancer Center fourth floor." The residents' pagers went off at the same time. They immediately stopped what they were doing and walked quickly out of the room. Not wanting to be left out, I followed them. I had no idea what I was doing or where I was going.

We arrived in the inpatient unit of the Karmanos Cancer Center. Our patient was an 89-year-old woman with stage IV lung cancer metastatic to her brain. She was thin, pale, and frail; her remaining vitality was consumed by the uncontrollable, rapidly dividing cancer cells. Her skin looked like white papier-mâché. The residents told me to "get in line for chest compressions." So I did.

I had practiced chest compressions on a mannequin, but this was my first time on a real person. When it was my turn, I was shocked how little resistance I encountered. I felt several popping sensations for the next 90 seconds as I manually pumped blood around her body. Suddenly, the residents pushed me away from the patient. I thought I had done something wrong, so I immediately apologized. The resident assertively said, "We have ROSC," pronounced "RAWsk." I learned later ROSC means "return of spontaneous circulation." Her heart started beating again.

That morning on rounds, the residents joked I had "the hands of God" and should be required to do chest compressions on all their patients. I didn't understand their comment, so our attending kindly explained chest compressions are not usually successful. A "code blue" means a patient's heart suddenly stopped. If a patient's heart suddenly stops inside of the hospital, there is a 75% chance they will not leave the hospital. Then my face turned red. I realized the residents were making fun of me! She politely told me I had been lucky.

Chest compressions are part of a larger strategy called cardiopulmonary resuscitation (CPR). If the heart stops for any reason, chest compressions should be started immediately so blood flow to the brain is not interrupted. My attending also explained the popping sounds—those were broken ribs. There is a common (and brutal) phrase in medical training when teaching chest compressions: "If you're not breaking ribs, you're not trying hard enough." This phrase exists because high-quality chest compressions are the most important factor for survival after cardiac arrest. Usually, a few broken ribs are preferential to hypoxic brain damage.[34]

Sometimes chest compressions aren't enough. Advanced cardiac life support (ACLS) is the medical management of life-threatening cardiovascular emergencies like heart attack, stroke, and cardiac arrest. ACLS is a way for strangers to coordinate effective emergency medical care within seconds of arriving at the bedside.

Algorithms are available for specific clinical situations such as cardiac arrest, low heart rate, and specific arrythmias. They all prioritize the heart because if the heart cannot pump blood, the brain cannot receive oxygen.[35]

---

34   A recent review of CPR is "In-Hospital Cardiac Arrest: A Review" written by Dr. Lars Anderson, published in the *Journal of the American Medical Association* in 2019. About 25% of in-hospital cardiac arrest patients survive to hospital discharge. Many are simply too old and too sick to survive. The woman described above passed away later the same day. Patients with reversible causes of cardiac arrest tend to do better than the 25% statistic.

35   The ACLS algorithms are available at acls.com/free-resources/acls-algorithms.

As a third-year medical student, I knew how to follow orders—that was it. I didn't realize it at the time, but in a few years I would be the one leading critical situations. That meant rapidly assessing the situation and then coordinating the correct management within seconds. At the time, I thought it was just following a protocol. Sounds simple enough, right?

§ PINK SHOES AND ICUS §

During my second call of intern year, I was on the surgical ward when two patients coded at the same time across the hall from each other. One was an elderly man who recently had a partial lung resection. He briefly lost pulses for an unknown reason. As I arrived at his room, another code was called across the hall. Multiple nurses asked rapid-fire questions as my pagers continued to go off. Drowning in pages with no idea what to do, I called the junior surgery resident for help. Even though she had multiple consults in the emergency department, she came to help me, her pink shoes moving at double speed.

She took one look at the patient, rapidly read his chart, gave direction to two nurses, and then made a phone call—all in the span of five minutes. She told me what happened, what to do about it, and then gave me the phone number of the surgical ICU. She had already diagnosed the patient, ordered the relevant labs and imaging, and arranged for an ICU bed. After that, she quickly dealt with the second code before I could type the surgical ICU phone number into my cell phone. *How was she so fast?*

She then circled back, gave me an empathetic look, and said, "One day, you will be in my shoes. Don't worry." Then she walked away at double speed back to the emergency department. I remember thinking, *Why would I want pink shoes?*

Eleven months later, I was again on call with the same junior surgery resident. I was paged by a nurse to see a colorectal surgery patient who had new difficulty breathing. Her respiratory rate was 45 breaths per minute and heart rate 140 beats per minute—both dangerously high and indicative of imminent cardiovascular collapse.

I arrived at the bedside, took one look at her, directed two nurses, then rapidly absorbed her medical history from the electronic medical record. I managed her hemodynamics, ordered the initial laboratory tests and imaging, and then arranged for her transfer to the surgical ICU. I presented the patient via phone to my junior resident. She said, "Sounds good. Now come to the ED. We have a trauma. I need your help."

This call was different from my prior call 11 months earlier. I diagnosed the patient with a pulmonary embolism. Because the patient could not have a CT scan for definitive diagnosis, the SICU team preemptively treated her. She slowly improved over the next week. A subsequent imaging study confirmed my initial diagnosis. Two weeks later, I saw the junior resident in the resident lounge. I told her about our first call and most recent one. I had come so far since the beginning of intern year! I thanked her for her patience and guidance over the last year. She awkwardly admitted she didn't remember our first call together.

Her face softened for a brief second, then quickly snapped back to her baseline serious look. Admittedly, my random expression of appreciation was a little embarrassing. Clearly, she had no time to join my feelings party. After an awkward silence, she told me about two patients I needed to follow up with after their surgeries earlier in the day. She told me to examine them, then call her with any problems. I never did buy pink shoes, but I did become better at managing cardiopulmonary emergencies.

Two years later, I was called to intubate an elderly man in the coronary care unit, an ICU for heart failure patients. He had an extensive medical history, including heart failure, kidney disease, sleep apnea, peripheral vascular disease, and pulmonary hypertension. The combination of his medical conditions meant small changes in his physiology would cause dangerous fluctuations in his vital signs. This was bad news for me because anesthetic drugs always cause changes in cardiac and pulmonary physiology.

At first, he was awake and talking. His breathing was not normal but also not critical. Initially, the ICU resident and I decided not to intubate him because the intubation could cause more harm than benefit. For now, he was struggling but still breathing on his own. Thirty minutes later, the ICU resident called again. Now he was barely arousable, likely rendered unconscious by excess carbon dioxide in his blood due to his inadequate respirations.

I knew he was at very high risk of deterioration, so I immediately directed the nurses to bring arterial and central venous catheter kits. I needed to place invasive lines to monitor his physiology. I quickly guided a hollow needle into his right femoral vein using anatomical landmarks. Then I threaded a flexible metal guidewire into his femoral vein, the first step in placing a central venous catheter.

I knew he could decompensate at any second, so I never took my hand off his femoral pulse. Before I could dilate his femoral vein to place the central venous catheter, his pulse disappeared. With one hand holding a wire in his femoral vein, I called a code blue.

I directed my junior resident to place a breathing tube while I led the nurses, respiratory therapists, and pharmacists in the proper ACLS protocols. During his nine minutes of high-quality chest compressions, he received epinephrine to raise his blood pressure and stimulate his heart, bicarbonate to buffer the acid in his blood, and multiple electric shocks for a deadly heart rhythm called ventricular fibrillation.

While directing the code, I managed to dilate his femoral vein and place the central venous catheter over the guidewire while nurses were doing chest compressions. After nine minutes, his heart restarted. We had ROSC. I had come a long way since my first day of residency. Perhaps I had learned something after all.

§ AIRWAY, BREATHING, CIRCULATION §

The ABCs of anesthesia are officially airway, breathing, and circulation. Unofficially, the ABCs are airway, bagel, coffee. Anesthesiologists love their bagels and coffee, but our specialty is actually about how to perfuse organs and tissues with oxygenated blood. Much of my training as an anesthesiologist is understanding how to resuscitate anyone, at any time, for any reason. Resuscitate means "return to physiologic stability."

We rarely think of the heart and lungs as essential organs because they are not consciously controlled. You don't tell your heart to beat or tell yourself to breathe; your brainstem controls both, without your conscious awareness. In fact, patients who suffer catastrophic neurologic injuries above the brainstem will continue to breathe spontaneously and have a heartbeat without any other neurologic function. We don't realize how important these essential functions are until a Black Swan occurs; then suddenly, they are the only things that matter.

When a crisis occurs, the most essential functions must be prioritized. This mode of thinking can be broadly applied if we think of the body as a complex system. When a medical complication crashes the body, anesthesiologists prioritize organs in a particular order to keep the patient alive long enough to locate and stop the synergistic interactions that created the complication.

All other organs and organ systems are dealt with only after the heart and lungs become functional again. You wouldn't want me as your doctor focusing on the sludge in your gallbladder when your heart stops, would you?

Prioritizing essential parts during emergencies is not unique to CPR and ACLS. Computers have preprogrammed contingency plans when they crash called RAS (reliability, availability, and serviceability). Hospitals have special red electrical outlets connected to backup generators in case of a sudden power grid failure. The most essential electrical components such as ventilators are plugged into these outlets for safety.

When emergency complications occur, priorities change to reflect the most essential parts of the system. Let's return to the case of the Black Swan called COVID-19.

§ SAVING THE GAUSSIAN PARTS §

When Black Swans occur, we can aid our decision making by separating complex systems into essential and synergistic categories. As described in Chapter 1, essential parts tend to be gaussian. They are bound by physical laws, amendable to direct measurement, and objective. Synergistic parts tend to be subjective, dependent on essential functions, and allow the system to complete more complicated tasks.

In terms of economics, the two interact in a symbiotic manner as pictured below.

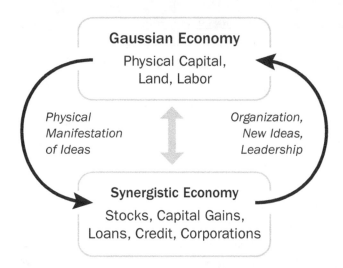

Gaussian Economy
Physical Capital,
Land, Labor

*Physical
Manifestation
of Ideas*

*Organization,
New Ideas,
Leadership*

Synergistic Economy
Stocks, Capital Gains,
Loans, Credit, Corporations

Figure 6-1

During a Black Swan, the valuable parts are overwhelmingly gaussian. Just as human ACLS focuses on the heart, lungs, and brain, economic ACLS should focus on resuscitating the gaussian parts. A new synergistic economy can grow from gaussian parts, but a new gaussian economy cannot grow from synergistic parts. An economy, just like a person, can be "rebooted" only from its gaussian parts.

For example, if a large airline company went bankrupt, what would happen? The legal entity would dissolve. Executives, administrators, and employees would lose their jobs. Investors would lose their stock. But there would still be a demand for air travel. Nothing can stop an entrepreneur from starting another airline company, buying the gaussian physical capital (planes, terminals, etc.), and employing the same workers.

On the flip side, if all pilots, flight attendants, and ground crews disappeared, no amount of synergistic management could build an airline company. Synergistic positions benefit in times of stability and, in exchange for that privilege, must be the first to be downsized in times in crisis.

In Part I, we covered the origins, observation, and psychology of synergy. In Part II, we discussed the management of Black Swans, including synergy monitors, managing the time horizon, and prioritizing resources. In Part III, we will focus on how anesthesiologists navigate specific characteristics of complex systems.

PART III

Characteristics of Complex Systems

CHAPTER 7

The Time Paradoxes

"You don't get another chance. Life is no Nintendo game!"
—EMINEM, "LOVE THE WAY YOU LIE"

"He who lives by the crystal ball soon learns to eat ground glass."
—EDGAR FIEDLER, AMERICAN ECONOMIST

Time only takes one path toward the future. In complex systems, there is no way to run the same experiment twice. If I give the same drug to the same patient at different times, the effect might be different. Blindly following patterns can lead to disastrous results, because every situation in a complex system is fundamentally unique. Even if one detail is different, that detail could be the difference between routine and a Black Swan.

In simple systems, time is irrelevant. I can redo the same math problem under the same circumstances as many times as I want until I solve it. If I'm playing a video game, I can redo the same level until I beat it. This doesn't represent reality, especially in complex systems with severe consequences for failure.

What if I treated my patients as simple experiments without regard to their safety? Would you want your doctor to do that? The first tenet of medicine is *primum non nocere*, "first, do no harm." Thriving in complex systems means accepting every situation is unique and approaching every one with the same vigilance as the previous. Every new event is an opportunity for success... and failure.

§ BIG KIDNEYS, BIG PROBLEMS §

I once had a patient with polycystic kidney disease. The disease is caused by mutations in cell signaling genes PKD1, PKD2, and PKD3, named for the disease in which the mutations occur (PKD stands for polycystic kidney disease). When the genes are defective, manifestations include widespread cyst formation in the kidneys, liver, and pancreas. It also causes weakening of blood vessel walls resulting in aortic and brain aneurysms.

The most recognized sign is enlarged, cystic, dysfunctional kidneys. If the kidneys become large enough, they can cause abdominal pain, acid reflux, and shortness of breath. My patient was a young man in his 30s with these exact symptoms. He was scheduled for robotic resection.[36]

Robotic urologic procedures are ominous for anesthesiologists. Greater than 99% of the time, they have no complications and the patients do well. But once in a while, a major blood vessel is injured, the bleeding cannot be controlled with the robotic arms,

---

36 There are three categories of abdominal surgery: open, laparoscopic, and robotic. Open means the surgeon can directly see your abdominal organs. Laparoscopic means the surgeon pumps gas into your abdomen and then performs surgery with long instruments through 1 cm incisions. One of those instruments is a camera that projects the abdominal cavity on a TV screen. Robotic surgery is similar to laparoscopic, but the instruments are controlled by a robotic interface. A surgeon then controls the robotic instruments like a video game. Robotic surgery is generally utilized for complicated or challenging operations.

and the patient bleeds out before an open surgical exploration can be done.

Large blood vessels like the renal artery, renal vein, inferior vena cava, and abdominal aorta can hemorrhage one liter of blood per minute. For perspective, the blood volume of a 70 kg person is about 5.5 L. Millimeters can be the difference between a successful surgery and massive hemorrhage. I'm always impressed my surgical colleagues don't injure *more* blood vessels. Their results are a testament to their precision.

On the morning of my patient's surgery, I induced anesthesia, then intubated uneventfully. The robot was docked and the urologists carefully dissected the fascial planes around the massive, cystic kidneys. During my residency, two patients died from vascular injuries during robotic urological surgery, so my eyes were glued to the video screen projecting the inside of the patient's abdomen. Thousands of robotic abdominal surgeries are done every year—the overall mortality rate is about 0.1%. I hoped this case would be in the uneventful 99.9%. Then I saw pulsating red liquid.[37]

In the next ten minutes, I gave him a liter of IV fluids. The surgeons quickly ligated the small bleeding artery. I breathed a sigh of relief. The rest of the surgery proceeded uneventfully. I extubated him in the OR, made sure he was breathing on his own, and then transported him to the post-anesthesia care unit (PACU) one floor below.

---

37 Mortality rates don't fully describe the risk of an individual surgery. Mortality reflects deaths from both surgical and nonsurgical causes. Surgical mortality for healthy patients is essentially nonexistent. A sick, chronically hospitalized patient is more likely to suffer complications than a healthy patient. So if a sick patient dies of a heart attack after a medically necessary surgery, the death is still counted as surgical mortality even if the cause of death is unrelated to the surgical procedure.

Upon arrival in the PACU three minutes later, a nurse plugged in his pulse oximeter. His oxygen saturation was 10%. I immediately ran to the bedside. He wasn't breathing. I quickly asked for an AMBU bag. As I watched his lips turn blue, I pushed oxygen into his lungs. His oxygen saturation slowly rose to 100% as the oxygen diffused from his lungs into his blood and circulated around his body.

The next 30 minutes were the scariest of my life. Even though only three minutes had passed since traveling from the OR to the PACU, I was still nervous. Hypoxic brain injury also only takes minutes. The only thing left to do was wait. As the anesthesia wore off, we would know if he had brain damage or not. After what seemed like an eternity, he woke up neurologically intact. I went into the hallway and paradoxically laughed with my head in my hands. I was less than a minute away from killing my patient.

As I talked with my attending (and several other attendings), we reviewed everything I did so I could learn from this complication. I certainly didn't want to make the same mistake again. I confirmed my patient was breathing before leaving the operating room, but looking back, I did a few things differently.

The operating room nurse was training a junior nurse, so I let her trainee push the gurney to the PACU; I usually drive to watch my patient's breathing. I asked the OR nurse if there was oxygen in the tank. She said yes, but I should have verified it for myself.

Perhaps the soft tissue of the mouth and pharynx collapsed and then prevented normal breathing. Anesthesiologists call this upper airway obstruction, but my patient was breathing appropriately when he left the OR. Perhaps there was no oxygen in the tank? Perhaps it wasn't turned on? Perhaps he simply obstructed, and I did not catch it because I didn't drive the bed?

I have taken thousands of patients to the PACU without this complication. Some I watched, some I didn't. Some I checked the oxygen tank myself, some I didn't. Most I drove, some I let my medical student or a nursing student drive. Where is the pattern? What could I have done differently?

Anesthesiology has changed significantly since the 1940s. Before pulse oximetry and capnography, anesthesiologists would literally watch their patients breathe. Barely perceptible changes in their chest excursion and breathing patterns were the only differences between waking up and permanent brain damage.

As I outlined earlier, modern anesthesia is safer than anesthesia in the 1940s due to anesthesiologists who know how to apply complex monitors and airway devices to ambiguous clinical situations. Some days, I feel like a modern anesthesiologist doing dangerous cases on complex patients with advanced monitors. Other days, I feel like an anesthesiologist in the 1940s, watching my patient breathe, praying he will wake up without brain damage.

Despite all my training I learned a valuable lesson that day: every situation is fundamentally unique even if they seem the same. The next day, I did a cardiac catheterization case on a pleasant man in his 80s. He was calm, kind, and grateful for the doctors and nurses—the ideal patient. The case was uneventful. He was extubated in the same manner as my polycystic kidney disease patient. He was also breathing on his own.

The nurses and I moved him from the OR bed to the gurney before transport to the PACU. I checked the oxygen tank. It was empty.

§ TIME §

Navigating simple and complex systems is fundamentally different. Complex systems like the operating room have an infinite scope and unclear cause and effect. Rules may be known or unknown, and feedback may or may not occur. This is in contrast to simple systems where cause and effect are immediately observable, rules are clear, feedback is immediate, and you know when you are correct or incorrect.

Differences are summarized below.

	SIMPLE SYSTEM	COMPLEX SYSTEM
CAUSE AND EFFECT	Easily seen	Often unclear
RULES	Clearly defined	Unknown
FEEDBACK	Immediate and timely	Delayed or absent
RANGE	Finite set of known complications	Infinite set of known and unknown complications
ACTIONS	Similar actions yield similar results	Similar actions yield different results
EXAMPLES	Math problems, video games, multiple-choice tests	Anesthesiology, COVID-19, economics

Figure 7-1

These differences occur because of time. Because time only flows in one direction, it introduces three paradoxes into simple system models of objective reality.

The first time paradox is events in the past change the future such that every new situation is unique. Unknown synergistic interactions between the first action and the complex system permanently change the complex system so the same action repeated multiple times acts on a unique system every time. I observed this in high school when the coolant reservoir of my car cracked in the middle of winter. Every time I drove my car, the plastic reservoir expanded and contracted due to temperature changes. Structural weaknesses developed, and eventually a single hot-cold cycle cracked the coolant reservoir. Suddenly, my car started smoking on the highway.

Surgeons see this same phenomenon in patients who have multiple abdominal surgeries. After every surgery, adhesions (bands of fibrous tissue) grow between abdominal organs and the abdominal wall. Every past surgery makes every future surgery different—and usually more difficult—than the previous one. Even though the patient may look the same, the outcome can be very different. If too many adhesions are present, sometimes an operation cannot be done safely.

Anesthesiologists see the same pattern in arteries and veins accessed multiple times. They scar down and then become more difficult to access in the future. Certain chronic medical conditions can also make veins more difficult to access over time. Interventions and complexity fundamentally change the system such that every subsequent intervention is fundamentally different from the previous one.

The second time paradox is events cannot be fully understood. After an intervention, there is no way to know all the synergistic interactions that occurred. I can't prove the crack in my coolant reservoir was caused by thermal expansion and contraction. Perhaps I drove over a pothole? Perhaps the part was faulty? Perhaps it was installed incorrectly? Perhaps another engine component malfunctioned causing an unavoidable problem with the coolant reservoir? I will never know.

I can't go back to my PKD patient and see what happened. Risk factors leading up to the event can be identified, and the results can be analyzed, but the exact mechanism of events cannot be determined. In a simple system, one action always yields a predictable result, but in a complex system, there is always uncertainty. If there was no uncertainty, there would be no complications, and because complications exist, we must assume some uncertainty is always present.

The third time paradox is mistakes are not always recognized when they occur. After a mistake is made, how do we know it was a mistake? You might not have noticed something that would have changed your decision, and you have no way to know about it. Navigating a complex system is like finding your way through an unfamiliar house in complete darkness. You never know if you will find the light switch. You might walk into a wall or stub your toe. Just be careful not to knock over a vase or break a TV. The difference is, in anesthesiology we don't break a vase; we kill our patient.

I will never know if my actions (or inaction) caused harm to my PKD patient. Perhaps I would have seen him stop breathing if I drove the bed? Perhaps the oxygen tank was not working correctly? Perhaps he would have stopped breathing regardless of my actions? There is no way for me to confirm causation after the event.

Perhaps I should just invent a time machine and save myself the headache.

§ INTERVIEWING IN TEXAS §

In complex systems, learning is not organized as it is in simple systems. There is no way to know ahead of time if a fact is useful or not. There are no chapters, syllabi, or classes. A single fact I learned a decade ago or a unique patient I saw in medical school might become suddenly applicable to a random future situation.

My mind must be organized in such a way to retrieve random memories at a moment's notice, then draw the correct connections between those memories and a new situation I have never seen before.

During my third year of residency, I traveled to Houston, Texas to the Texas Heart Institute to interview for a critical care fellowship. Because the current fellow giving me a tour was on call that day, I went with him to the surgical ICU for a possible intubation.

Our patient was a healthy 65-year-old man who developed a large sarcoma (cancer of connective tissue) in his abdomen. After an exploratory laparotomy (large midline incision), the cancer was resected, and then a transversus abdominis plane (TAP) block was performed by the anesthesiologist. TAP blocks numb the nerves of the abdominal wall for better pain control. They are especially useful for large abdominal incisions.

The patient had received a small dose (0.6 mg) of the IV pain medication hydromorphone (trade name Dilaudid) four hours earlier. Clinically, the effects of hydromorphone typically last between two and four hours. But now he was in the ICU, barely breathing enough to stay awake. He was completely unresponsive.

The ICU team asked for an anesthesiologist consultation before intubation. I went with the fellow to assess the patient. No one understood why he was so obtunded. The dose of pain medication given to him in the operating room was too small and too far in the past to cause this degree of somnolence. Usually, a patient would need between 2 mg and 4 mg within 30 minutes to be that "zonked."

I suggested we give the patient naloxone (trade name Narcan), a medication that reverses opioids like hydromorphone. Everyone else in the room was skeptical—a small amount of IV pain medication given four hours prior would not cause his symptoms. But I insisted. After a few minutes of discussion, the nurse reluctantly gave 0.1 mg of naloxone. Nothing happened.

Then I asked her to give more; 0.2 mg was given. No effect. More; 0.5 mg. No effect. Then I asked her to give the entire 1 mg. She looked very uncomfortable as she emptied the syringe into the patient. Suddenly, he woke up, took a deep breath, opened his eyes, and asked where he was. Everyone stared at me. I smiled.

After he woke up, I explained myself. During a Sunday night general surgery call of my intern year, I was doing post-operative checks on the surgical patients admitted to the floor that day. I remember one patient who was sleeping comfortably despite a large abdominal incision. Strangely, he had not requested any pain medication.

The nurse shrugged and said he had some kind of nerve block. I called the regional anesthesiology fellow and asked about the block. Apparently, the patient received a TAP block in the operating room after surgery. The fellow laughed and said, "It must be one hell of a TAP block! Guess who did it? Yeah, that's right—me!"[38]

A random phone call years ago gave me the exact answer to an

---

38 Regional anesthesiology is a subspecialty of anesthesiology specializing in peripheral nerve blocks. More information can be found at asra.com or nysora.com.

unpredictable future problem. A few months after my visit to the Texas Heart Institute, I was offered an ICU fellowship. I graciously accepted.

§ ACCEPTING RESPONSIBILITY §

The standard of practice in a complex system is perfection. Nature does not give out participation medals. The difference between success and failure can be as nuanced as letting a nursing student push the bed or seeing an unusual TAP block several years ago.

In anesthesiology, our patients cannot maintain their own vital functions, which means if I do not recognize an error, my patient can die within minutes. I need to recognize any problem occurring at any time for any reason.

The responsibility is both exciting and terrifying. Every time I induce anesthesia, I'm both confident I can deal with all the complications and scared I will overlook a small detail and accidentally kill my patient. Being an anesthesiologist is living a double life— one self has the cool confidence to domesticate nature, and the other lives in crippling paranoia.

There is a certain satisfaction of transporting fellow humans to the brink of death, keeping them in a state of suspended animation, then delivering them back to life. But there is also fear. Despite all of my near misses, I have not lost a patient in my care—yet. The day may come that I have one unrecognized complication resulting in a patient death. So far, I have proven my ability to rescue myself from emergency situations, but one day, fortune may not be on my side.

As I prepare to leave residency, this weight weighs heavy on my shoulders. Soon I will assume sole responsibility for my clinical decisions. My attitude toward this responsibility has also changed. Much of my training as a physician has been understanding how to sort through ambiguity, to make the unseen seen, and the unknown known.

Now I realize my future will require me to live with increasing amounts of ambiguity. I will be the one to make life-or-death decisions for another human being, and I will have no one to tell me if I was right or wrong. The world will transition from black and white into shades of gray.

I find myself with a massive responsibility ahead and no way back to simpler times. Becoming a physician is a permanent, life-altering decision. My friends and family ask me questions about their medical problems. If someone experiences a medical emergency, I am obligated to help them. By accepting that responsibility, I am also accepting the responsibility to do that work well. The lives of my patients will be decided by how I interpret complexity and ambiguity.

On a larger scale, the time paradoxes will play an even greater role as our world becomes more complex. Despite the increasing ambiguity, we will still have to make decisions every day. The *choice* to accept the responsibility is not really a *choice*. By enjoying the benefits of complexity, we have already accepted the responsibility to take care of it. Our future is in our hands whether we like it or not. We cannot change the progression of time, but we can learn to factor it into our decisions to achieve better outcomes.

In the next chapter, we will continue looking at the characteristics of complex systems. We will be better prepared to navigate them by understanding how synergy changes over time, a characteristic called propagation.

CHAPTER 8

Propagation

"The best physicians recognize their complications before their patient is harmed. Beware those who have no complications."

—Physician proverb

"Fate is like a strange, unpopular restaurant filled with odd little waiters who bring you things you never asked for and don't always like."

—Lemony Snicket, author of *A Series of Unfortunate Events*

When I was shadowing my family physician in my fourth year of undergrad, I came across an interesting patient. He was a kind, middle-aged gentleman with a wife and two adult children. He worked for a bottling company delivering water and pop to various businesses in southeastern Michigan. Overall, he described his life as happy. He had a wonderful family, financial stability, and plenty of time to pursue personal interests outside of work. He was also addicted to narcotics.[39]

His drug of choice was an opioid called oxycodone. Opioids are

---

39 I grew up in Michigan where we call carbonated sugary beverages pop. When I moved to Los Angeles, those same beverages became soda. Apparently, in the South they are called coke, which is apparently different from Coca-Cola.

analgesics (drugs that relieve pain) that act in the brain and spinal cord. In the early 1800s, the first opiate was isolated in Germany. It was named morphine after Morpheus, the Greek god of sleep. Since then, stronger opioids have been designed in chemistry laboratories, including oxycodone.[40]

His addiction started when he hurt his back several years ago and was prescribed oxycodone. The correct clinical management should have been rest, stretching, physical therapy, and NSAIDs (nonsteroidal anti-inflammatory drugs like ibuprofen) rather than opioids.[41]

Narcotics often cause temporary euphoria when given inappropriately, contributing to their addictive potential. After his prescription ran out, he started buying oxycodone and other unknown narcotics from drug dealers. His life collapsed. He was fired from his job. His wife threatened divorce. His kids stopped talking to him. Eventually, he went to rehab, repaired his relationships, and got his life back.

Even though he was no longer taking street drugs, the opioid addiction permanently changed his brain chemistry. He will be at high risk of relapse for the rest of his life. To prevent further complications, he now takes a medication called buprenorphine supervised by a physician.

---

40 Narcotic, opiate, and opioid are technically different. Narcotic is a legal term referring to a controlled substance frequently abused outside of its appropriate therapeutic purpose. Opiate is a scientific term referring to naturally occurring analgesics found in nature that bind to a specific class of pain receptors in the brain. Opioids are derivatives of opiates synthesized in a chemistry laboratory.

41 Opioids for back pain may be indicated in specific situations, but generally, they are not the first-line treatment. Every opioid prescription carries a risk of addiction. The treatment of back pain should focus on treating the cause of the pain rather than masking its symptoms.

Buprenorphine is a partial opioid agonist, meaning it stimulates the opioid receptors just enough to prevent addictive cravings but doesn't cause euphoria. He takes a small dose every day and checks in with his physician every month to make sure he is doing well. I would never guess the kind, calm, rational man in front of me was at one time in his life addicted to drugs.

Was his addiction 100% his fault? The easy answer is, he made all those choices and should be responsible for them. But the correct answer is more complicated.

Addiction *rarely* appears out of nowhere; knowable and unknowable risk factors are usually present. The cause of addiction is often multifactorial, including genetic, psychological, and environmental factors. Addiction runs in families. Genetically inherited brain chemistry probably plays a role. Certain personality types are also more prone to addictive behaviors. Environment plays a role, as addiction is more common when additive substances are readily available. Some people are simply more susceptible to addiction, and when they are given highly addictive substances without their knowledge, it is like lighting a fire in a field of dry brush.

This was the first time I recognized propagation, when a single uncorrected mistake causes exponentially more mistakes over time. In simple systems, there is immediate feedback like checking the answer key after a math problem. Therefore, one mistake *decreases* the likelihood of a future mistake.

However, complex systems do not have answer keys. Mistakes *increase* the likelihood and intensity of future mistakes. Propagation exists because components of a complex system can interact with each other to create additional events. If these interactions are not controlled, they will eventually organize into Black Swans.

Below are diagrams of error propagation in simple and complex systems.

Simple system:

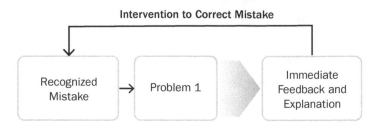

Figure 8-1

Complex system:

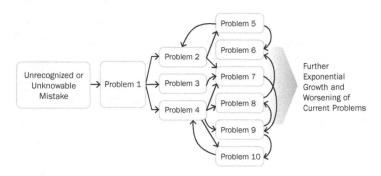

Figure 8-2

The damage done to a complex system can take years to fix or be permanent. This man was lucky he went to rehab before his wife divorced him or he ended up dead.

§ THE FIFTH VITAL SIGN §

In 1995, Dr. James Campbell, in his address to the American Pain Society, urged pain to be treated as a "fifth vital sign" along with heart rate, blood pressure, temperature, and respiratory rate. This is the origin of the 1–10 pain scale commonly used in clinical practice.

At the time, this logic made sense: uncontrolled, acute pain can cause a multitude of poor medical outcomes and poor quality of life. Nurses were encouraged to treat pain more aggressively, doctors were encouraged to make pain medication more available, and some financial reimbursement from Medicare was tied to pain control. At the same time, an opportunistic marketing campaign for a drug called oxycodone was launched by Purdue Pharma; it advocated opioids as a means to meet these new goals.

The quest to treat pain without understanding its source resulted in the opioid crisis, a name for the propagation of synergistic damage caused by overprescribing opioids. This crisis includes medical complications of abuse compounded by the difficulty of rehabilitating addicts, social costs of drug abuse, lost productivity, and at least 40,000 deaths per year. In my fourth year of medical school, I spent a month conducting autopsies at the Wayne County Coroner's Office in Detroit, Michigan. Half of our "patients" were opioid overdoses.[42]

Twenty-five years later, physicians have a different perspective of pain management. During my residency, I received special instruction in the treatment of acute and chronic pain with both medications and interventional procedures.

Anesthesiologists are most qualified to treat pain; we do it every

---

42 A brief summary of the opioid crisis is "Enduring Pain: How a 1996 Opioid Policy Change Had Long-Lasting Effects" by Edward Helmore, published in *The Guardian*. A comprehensive summary is "The Opioid Crisis: A Comprehensive Overview" by Nalili Vadivelu, published in an academic journal called *Current Pain and Headache Reports*.

day in the operating rooms, labor and delivery, and outpatient pain clinics. Treating pain appropriately to avoid synergistic propagation is a combination of understanding its complex origins, managing patient expectations, and controlling the possible synergistic effects of the available treatment regimens.

Sometimes pain is related to a physical stimulus—such as a surgeon's knife—and other times it has no physical stimulus at all. Overtreating pain with opioids can alter pain receptors in the brain and spinal cord causing hyperalgesia (pain out of proportion to physical stimuli) and addiction. Undertreating pain increases the risk of acute pain converting to chronic pain.

Chronic pain can develop when uncontrolled pain permanently activates neurons in the spinal cord and brain to give the sensation of pain even after the physical source no longer exists. Diagnosis and treatment is further complicated by how people cope with adversity, their psychological profile, and their genetics.

Because synergy is not directly measurable, propagation usually goes unrecognized until its effects are perceived indirectly. No one can know the moment when a person becomes addicted to opioids, but we can observe unusual behavior. Sometimes addiction takes years to be recognized and even longer to be corrected. In the meantime, the disease causes widespread damage and chaos. Without intervention, the damage will become irreversible.

Below is a graph describing propagation of synergy over time. The X-axis represents time and the Y-axis synergy, and the curve represents synergistic propagation. The dashed lines indicate the perception threshold where synergistic effects are first noticed and the point at which irreversible damage occurs.

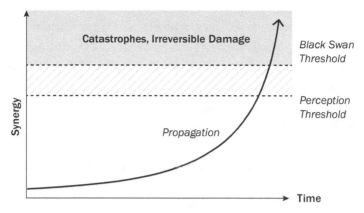

Figure 8-3

In this specific case, the inciting event is an opioid prescription, the propagation is addiction, and the perception threshold is self-destructive behaviors. Catastrophic Black Swans are permanent consequences, such as death or permanent disability.

§ A MORE COMPLEX PATIENT §

The more complex a system is, the faster synergy propagates. For the first patient, harmful synergy was extinguished before permanent damage occurred. In his case, synergistic complications were recognized and the source of his problem was addressed. He was relatively simple compared to our next patient.

I met her the morning after she had surgery for stomach cancer. At the time, she took 120 mg of morphine per day, enough to sedate an elephant. Because she chronically took a high dose of opioids, she was exquisitely sensitive to painful sensations, but pain medications had little analgesic effect. However, she was still vulnerable to the side effects of those medications, including respiratory depression.[43]

---

43 The usual starting dose is 5–10 mg for an adult.

On the surgical ward, she was given so much IV opioid pain medication that her respiratory rate dropped to zero. One minute she was in 10/10 pain and screaming; the next, she wasn't breathing. A code blue was called, then a breathing tube was inserted, and she was promptly revived. She arrived in the ICU with a few broken ribs. That's where I met her.[44]

I managed her care in the ICU for the next week. She was a clever, Caucasian woman in her 50s. Contrary to my initial expectations, she was very intelligent. Her hair was bushy like Hermione Granger from the Harry Potter series. I could tell she was used to negotiating in order to get her way. Later, I learned she used to be a lawyer.

After we removed the breathing tube, she constantly demanded more pain medications no matter how much we gave her. Eventually, she was transferred to the floor where she developed a severe bowel obstruction most likely due to chronic opioid use. A single surgery kept her in the hospital for more than a month due to complications related to opioids.

The next month, I saw her multiple times on the inpatient pain service. She was unofficially my "personal patient" because I knew her well and no one else wanted to deal with her demands. Over time, she and I found common ground. I learned about her past law career, addiction struggles, current frustrations in the hospital, and hopes for the future.

She had lost her friends, family, job, and financial independence. In turn, we formed a constructive relationship based on respect,

---

44 This is how opioid addicts accidentally commit suicide. They require higher and higher doses to achieve the same euphoria. Eventually, they take a high enough dose to make them stop breathing. Then they slowly suffocate in their drug-induced stupor.

clear expectations, and honest communication. With time, like our relationship, her condition improved. Once I even saw her at the hospital Starbucks casually ordering coffee.

Chronic pain patients are often misunderstood. Their pain is not taken seriously because it seems out of proportion to their physical symptoms. They are often labeled "difficult" because they are constantly asking for pain medications. They experience more complications than patients without chronic pain because every part of their medical care is affected by their pain.

Pain is difficult to treat because it can't be directly measured; it is a subjective representation of suffering. Furthermore, pain is influenced by the context in which it occurs. It cannot be *truly* defined or standardized.

The second patient was much more complex, synergy propagated faster, and she experienced more complications compared to the first patient. The difference in their outcomes highlights the difference between propagation in a simple system (mistake recognized quickly, then treated before irreversible damage occurred) versus propagation in a complex system (synergy quickly causing irreversible damage and increased risk of Black Swans).

§ PROPAGATION AND COVID-19 §

Very complex systems distort cause-and-effect relationships because a single action, in addition to its direct effects, causes hidden random synergistic interactions. Those systems, such as the second patient, have a long lag time followed by a rapid increase in synergy. By the time the complications are recognized, it is too late; synergy is dangerously high and already producing Black Swans. The two models are shown below.

Simple system:

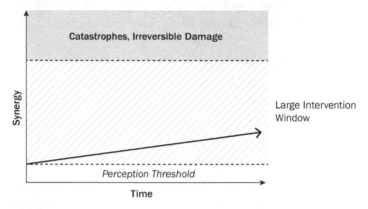

Figure 8-4

Simple systems do not have lag time because their effects are immediately recognized. The intervention window is large because synergy does not functionally exist.

Complex system:

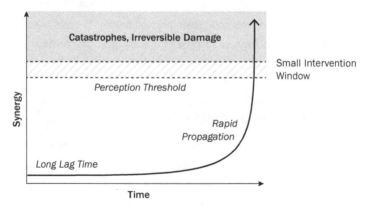

Figure 8-5

Complex systems exhibit lag time, rapid progression, and a small opportunity for intervention. As complexity increases, lag time increases, the rate of rapid propagation increases, and the opportunity for intervention decreases. We see an example of this with SARS-CoV-2. SARS-CoV-2 is highly synergistic: it has a long lag time, rapid propagation, and a small intervention window.[45]

The lag time for COVID-19 exists for two reasons: lack of a perfect diagnostic test and delayed symptom onset. First, COVID-19 PCR tests (mouth/nasopharyngeal swab) are not 100% accurate. The sensitivity varies between 30% and 90% depending on the time since symptom onset. This means at least 10% of the time, the test will be negative when the person is actually infected by SARS-CoV-2. If both asymptomatic and symptomatic spreaders exist, how do we know who has the disease and who doesn't?[46]

Second, the symptoms of the disease appear between two and four days after infection. By the time the infected person knows he or she is infected, he or she probably already spread the disease to others, if the person even knew at all. Additionally, how are government officials supposed to know what to do if we don't know where the virus is or who is spreading it? The disease spread is not perceptible, so it appears to have a lag time.

---

45 SARS-CoV-2 refers to the virus itself: SARS stands for "severe acute respiratory syndrome," CoV stands for "coronavirus," and 2 refers to this coronavirus as the second one to cause a severe acute respiratory illness in humans. The first one occurred between 2002 and 2004 and was simply called SARS. COVID-19 refers to the constellation of symptoms caused by SARS-CoV-2. COVID stands for "coronavirus disease" and the 19 stands for 2019, the year it was first reported.

46 The sensitivity and positive predictive value of the COVID PCR test is currently being studied. As of 2021, the sensitivity is about 70%, meaning the test will be falsely negative about 30% of the time. An academic summary of the PCR test is "Clinical Sensitivity and Interpretations of PCR and Serological COVID-19 Diagnostics for Patients Presenting to the Hospital" by Dr. Tyler Miller published in *The Journal of the Federation of American Societies for Experimental Biology* in August 2020.

The effect of interventions occurs approximately two weeks later because people take about two weeks to recover from the disease. The prolonged disease duration allows confounding factors to mask the true cause-and-effect relationships of our interventions.

Rapid propagation can also be seen in COVID-19. As the virus spreads throughout a population, more and more people require hospitalization. Finally, the effects can be perceived but still seem small relative to the true burden of the disease. Then more people are infected. Finally, hospitals start filling up. A 30% COVID-19 hospital occupancy rate is much more than three times worse than a 10% occupancy rate. The risk profile increases exponentially rather than linearly.

Eventually, hospitals will fill up. At this point, Black Swans will fracture our healthcare infrastructure: elective surgeries will be canceled, ambulances will have nowhere to bring patients, and essential resources such as masks and oxygen become scarce. Additional people will die because they cannot receive the medical care they need. Once a COVID-19 outbreak reaches a critical level, it is too late. Southern California reached this point in December 2020. At one point my co-residents and I were intubating ten COVID patients *per day*.

The synergistic spread of SARS-CoV-2 seems to mirror its physiologic mechanism of disease. The virus causes a massive storm of cell signaling molecules called cytokines. Cytokine release occurs in an exponential manner: one molecule stimulates cells to release five more, then those five molecules stimulate 25 more, then 125, and so on. Doctors call a massive, unregulated release of cytokines "cytokine storm."

Cytokine storm causes massive inflammation that damages all

organs of the body, including the brain, heart, lungs, kidneys, and intestines. By the time this massive inflammatory reaction occurs, it cannot be stopped. Black Swan events, such as heart attack, stroke, pulmonary embolism, and acute respiratory distress syndrome destroy the infrastructure of the human body.

Although the mortality rate is 1%, patients can suffer lasting damage to their essential organs. As time goes on, more and more survivors will accumulate chronic medical problems from the disease. These chronic illnesses will increase the propagation speed of future medical complications just as my second patient's chronic opioid use increased the speed and severity of her medical complications. Synergy begets synergy.

§ HIDDEN LIABILITIES EVERYWHERE §

COVID-19 takes advantage of a blind spot in human psychology: we tend to believe our world behaves as a simple system when in reality it behaves like a complex system. We overestimate what we do know and underestimate what we don't know. This false approximation of reality causes people to downplay factors they don't fully understand.

Anesthesiologists take the opposite approach: we manage situations based on what we don't know rather than what we do know. We assume our world looks more like a complex system from the beginning.

In the operating room, I make simple, small, constant upstream modifications to a patient's anesthetic to control the synergy of the system. Anesthesiologists want to be bored because that means synergy is well controlled. Our specialty prefers to take the fewest actions possible. We do this because the more complex a patient, the more likely one action can accidentally propagate large synergistic changes. And for us, large synergistic changes dramatically increase the likelihood of patient death.

Anesthesiology is understanding the difference between harmful, inconsequential, and beneficial synergy. We must know what abnormal vital signs and lab values require intervention and which ones can be tolerated. Outside the range of normal does not always mean disease causing. Some blood pressures that are dangerous for one patient are safe for another. Sometimes a low pulse oximeter reading is a false positive. Every change in heart rate does not need to be treated with medication. The longer I practice, the more I realize the answer to most questions is, it *depends*. Sometimes the best course of action is to do nothing. Every intervention has side effects.

In fact, interventions can cause more complications than they fix. Doctors call the harm caused by their good-intentioned actions *iatrogenesis*. Anesthesiologists aim to optimize beneficial synergy while minimizing iatrogenic injury. Chapter 9 will continue the exploration of iatrogenesis.

CHAPTER 9

Iatrogenesis

"Really successful people say no to almost everything."

—WARREN BUFFETT

"Give the laziest person the most difficult job and he will find the most efficient way to do it."

—CALEB NORGAARD

A classic example of iatrogenesis is called the "cobra effect," named after a famous anecdote from colonial India. The story goes something like this:

> "In Colonial India, the British decided there were too many cobras in Delhi, so they offered a monetary reward for every dead cobra. Some enterprising Indian citizens decided to farm cobras to make money. Eventually, the British realized what was happening, so they rescinded the reward. The cobra farmers, without a financial incentive to breed cobras, released the snakes into the city. Now Delhi had a worse cobra problem than before."[47]

---

47   I first heard of the cobra effect from episode #96 of Freakonomics radio.

The cobra effect describes a strategy that works in theory but backfires in reality. Iatrogenesis is from the Greek words *iatros* meaning "healer" and *genesis* meaning "origin." It literally means "originating from the healer." For the purpose of this book, it will be defined as "an action meant to solve a problem that creates additional unintended consequences."

Much of my role in the operating room is minimizing the iatrogenic complications of my own actions. In anesthesiology, doing as little as possible is a virtue, not a vice. Action always invokes a penalty. Thinking is free. Choosing the incorrect action has a double penalty; you create more complications AND give up the opportunity to find the correct solution.

Anesthesiology is like living in the Old Testament: every mistake is harshly punished, and there is no such thing as redemption. To make matters worse, there is no time to consult other physicians when a complication occurs. Because complications rapidly propagate into Black Swans, anesthesiologists must think through the risks and benefits of every part of their anesthetic. Sometimes additional action without clear benefit is not worth the risk, especially when the minimum acceptable outcome is perfection.

Favorable outcomes in complex systems mean making as few moves as possible to achieve a desired outcome because this decreases the potential for iatrogenic harm. The first part of the chapter will cover complications from routine procedures, then we will discuss the "time penalty," and finally cover harm caused by incorrect interventions. We will see how choosing the correct intervention at the right time is more difficult than it seems. Every intervention, even when indicated, can cause negative synergistic consequences.

§ NO SUCH THING AS ROUTINE §

Every action has the potential for iatrogenic complications. Even commonly performed procedures, such as central lines, can result in significant patient harm. A central line (aka central venous catheter) is a large IV placed in one of the large veins leading to the heart. They are used to give large amounts of fluids (up to 500 cc/min), vasoactive medications (raise and lower blood pressure), medications too irritating for peripheral veins (such as chemotherapy and IV nutrition), or to measure the central venous pressure (provide information about cardiac function and fluid balance). When I was a third-year medical student, they seemed like a common, benign procedure.

This all changed during my fourth year of medical school when I observed an abnormal central line on one of my critical care rotations. The central line was supposedly placed in the subclavian vein, just below the collarbone. However, the pressure measured by the line was 128/64, consistent with the subclavian artery! When I discovered it in the morning before rounds, I immediately called the critical care fellow. He immediately called for a vascular surgery consultation. The surgeons immediately booked her for emergency surgery.

If the subclavian artery is accidentally dilated during central line placement, the catheter cannot simply be pulled out; the hole in the artery will continue to bleed until the patient dies. Vascular surgeons must surgically explore the area, fix the hole, then if necessary, repair the surrounding structures.

As my residency progressed, I saw other complications of central lines. Once I was called to emergently intubate a surgical ICU patient in liver failure waiting for a liver transplant offer. A central line was placed in her neck earlier that day without any initial complications.

Slowly over the course of the day, the right side of her neck expanded. She developed a hematoma at the entry site. Eventually, it grew large enough to cause shortness of breath. It was compressing her trachea. Now she had to be intubated before the hematoma completely occluded her airway.

Due to her advanced liver disease, unstable vital signs, and expanding hematoma, I needed to perform an awake fiberoptic intubation, where a thin flexible scope with a camera on the end is guided past the tongue and into the trachea while the patient is fully awake. By the time I arrived, her trachea was deviated toward the left side. Her heart rate was 140 and respiratory rate was 30. The hematoma was expanding every hour.

Despite the chaos around me, I patiently anesthetized her airway with numbing medication, then carefully directed the scope around her distorted anatomy past her vocal cords, and slid the endotracheal tube into place, as her oxygen saturation plummeted. Then I removed the scope and gently ventilated her. There were no complications. She eventually received a liver transplant and left the hospital two months later.

Other complications I have personally seen include collapsed lungs, arrythmias, and once a central line accidentally lodged in the chest millimeters away from the heart. Every action has a potential price. Luckily, I have avoided complications with central lines…so far.

I am meticulous when inserting central lines even on uncomplicated patients. Everything must be perfect every time. The cost of taking extra precautions is less than the cost of increasing the risk of complications. There is no way to measure the number of complications I prevented by choosing the correct site, correct patient, or using the correct technique.

Sometimes the best course of action is *not* placing a central line because something more important should be done first. When no complications occur, a central line placed at the correct time invokes only the penalty of the time spent doing it. However, if it is placed at the wrong time, it invokes a double penalty: both the potential complications from its placement and the opportunity cost of the time itself.

§ CRANIOTOMIES §

As an intern on general surgery call, I saw an elderly Persian woman who was run over by a bus. She was emergently intubated, then taken to the CT scanner to find all her fractures. Among other injuries, her jaw was broken, her skull was cracked, and she had bleeding in her brain.

Active bleeding in the brain is a surgical emergency. The neurosurgeons booked her for a craniotomy, literally *crani* referring to the skull and *otomy* a Latin term meaning "to create a hole in something." As an intern, my job was to help any way I could, so I went with her to the ICU in order to place arterial and central lines.

I suctioned blood from her mouth, presumably from her jaw fractures, as other residents placed the lines. She spent an extra hour in the ICU due to transportation delays. I continued to suction blood from her mouth. After two hours, I had 350 cc, about the volume of a pop can.

Eventually, she was taken to the operating room, and her skull was opened. The neurosurgeons worked efficiently to find the source of the bleeding. Blood kept coming out of the patient's mouth. Despite the successful surgical intervention, the patient's vital signs continued to deteriorate. Ten seconds after the surgeons closed her scalp, her heart stopped.

The surgeons quickly removed the surgical drapes, and then I started chest compressions. She was ice cold. I noticed grapefruit-sized hematomas in her groins where the central line and arterial line were placed. Blood continued to flow freely from her mouth. Despite 20 units of blood products (about 7 L), 30 minutes of chest compressions, and ACLS, she never regained pulses. She was dead. I looked down at my pager: I had 20 messages waiting.

The trauma Triad of Death is coagulopathy, hypothermia, and acidosis.[48] All three are caused by and contribute to bleeding. Acidosis and hypothermia prevent the biochemical reactions of the body from working correctly because the reactions are pH and temperature dependent. Coagulopathy is worsened by bleeding, hypothermia, and acidosis. The presence of one of the factors increases the likelihood of the others, which then increases the likelihood of further decompensation. The three act in synergistic fashion to propagate life-threatening hemorrhage.

If the Triad becomes uncontrollable, the patient cannot be saved. This patient had bled too much, was too cold, and was too acidotic. Perhaps I should have spoken up sooner—the excessive bleeding from her mouth was a telltale sign the Triad was propa-

---

48 Coagulopathy means impaired blood clotting. Hypothermia means abnormally low temperature. Acidosis in this context means the tissues of the body are not receiving enough oxygen, so instead of aerobic metabolism (using oxygen), they resort to less efficient anaerobic metabolism (without oxygen). Anaerobic metabolism produces more acid, which then propagates the original Triad.

gating faster than we thought. Her time in the ICU likely cost her her life. She should have been in the operating room immediately so the source of her blood loss could be addressed. Despite the perfectly executed surgery, we were too late.

Two years later, I was on an anesthesiology call when my pager went off around 2:00 a.m. A young man needed an emergency craniotomy after a motorcycle accident. I called the emergency department and surgery resident and specifically directed them not to waste any time. The patient should be sent to the operating room immediately. No central or arterial lines were to be placed in the emergency department. The patient should not be sent to the ICU before the OR.

I briskly walked to the eighth floor to set up the operating room. A nurse and surgical tech were already there opening sterilized surgical instruments. I drew up presser medications such as norepinephrine and vasopressin, called the blood bank for additional blood products, and stocked up on ACLS drugs. Another anesthesiology resident joined me. The patient arrived before I was ready. Perfect timing.

We quickly induced anesthesia and gave him as much blood as we could push into his peripheral IVs. I placed an arterial line under the blue drapes as the surgeons cut through his scalp to access his skull. When they opened his skull, blood flooded onto the floor. His blood pressure bottomed out as the surgeons' feet were covered in blood.

The neurosurgery residents didn't flinch or hesitate for a second. They spent the next hour systematically locating and cauterizing the bleeding vessels while I transfused additional blood products to prevent coagulopathy and gave presser medications to maintain the patient's blood pressure. Eventually, the bleeding slowed down, his presser requirements decreased, and his blood pressure improved. The surgeons closed his skull, and then he was sent to the neurosurgical ICU to recover. He left the hospital one month later.

The operating room trains anesthesiologists to recognize potential problems early and then aggressively prevent their propagation. My early recognition of the trauma Triad of Death resulted in a favorable outcome. A few phone calls made early in the process prevented the Triad's synergistic propagation. Once a Black Swan occurs, even the correct intervention might not be enough to stop it. Prevention, on the other hand, never occurs too early.

Simple systems favor a single success at the price of many errors because in simple systems errors have no cost. A discussion of risks and benefits is not necessary. The strategy of "throw everything at the wall and see what sticks" breaks down in complex systems because of the time paradoxes, propagation, and iatrogenesis. In complex systems, errors have grave consequences. You pay dearly for your mistakes and are only awarded with survival if you succeed.

§ LESS IS MORE §

The first tenet of medicine is *primum non nocere*, Latin for "first, do no harm." Doctors do best by their patients when they focus on not harming them rather than helping them. Good-intentioned intervention without a reason is more likely to cause iatrogenic injury than provide benefits.

At this point in my training, I see how every drug I give and every line I place has potential consequences. Every time I take an action, I am incurring a risk of complications and a time opportunity cost.

When I started residency four years ago, I thought a physician should always be busy, doing everything he could to help his patients. Now I see the truth: that my potential to harm patients often exceeds my ability to help them. Being busy is not the same thing as being effective. Instead, I view my patients holistically, decide what needs to be done, and do it in the safest and most efficient manner possible. In the complex world, less is more.

Quality anesthesiology is supposed to be boring. Because we don't waste time chasing self-inflicted iatrogenic complications, we can pay attention to the rest of the room and plan accordingly. We remain preventative rather than reactionary. I spend my time in the operating room listening, thinking, and acting—in that order. Every surgeon knows a frantic anesthesiologist means something bad is about to happen.

In high-synergy scenarios, we strive to create as much boredom as possible because that gives us the opportunity to notice signs of propagation. Anesthesiologists learn to function in this way because we have nowhere to hide when we make a mistake. We can't consult another physician to share the blame. We can't blame the patient for not following directions. In the operating room, there is no diffusion of responsibility; there is only personal liability.

At the statistical (simple) level, every patient is an identical data point, but at the individual (complex) level, they are infinitely unique. One detail can void an established pattern. In psychology, this is called the "broken leg problem." A statistical formula may correctly predict the probability of a person going to the movies on a given day, but if I know that person has a broken leg, I can always beat the formula. Lifesaving clinical decisions require thinking rather than blindly following guidelines.

Anesthesiologists cannot hide their failures behind oversimplified theories about how the world should work. For the last 80 years, our habits were formed by direct observation of complex systems rather than abstract academic theories based on simple system models. Every day, I am forced to see reality for what it is, not what I want it to be. Anesthesiologists don't bother proving abstract theories. Instead, we invest our time into achieving excellent outcomes in objective reality.

We've now covered how to think about complex systems and synergy (Part I), how to manage Black Swans (Part II), and the unique phenomena observed in complex systems, such as the time paradoxes, propagation, and iatrogenesis (Part III).

In the final part of the book, we will explore concrete ways anesthesiologists overcome these difficulties to achieve their excellent results.

PART IV

Managing Complex Systems

CHAPTER 10

Skin in the Game

"Avoid taking advice from someone who gives advice for a living. Unless there is a penalty for that advice."

—Nassim Taleb

"Accountability is the most potent form of morality."

—Anonymous

Physicians are unique among healthcare professionals in that our actions are directly tied to the legal definition of our personhood. Nurses, respiratory therapists, and NPPs (nonphysician providers) generally act under the direction of a physician. They do not have a medical education and therefore cannot be personally responsible for their actions. They can be fired, but they generally do not suffer additional legal consequences if they are employed by another legal entity, such as a hospital.[49]

Physicians, however, can be personally sued if they practice below

49 NPPs include nurse practitioners, physician assistants, and nurse anesthetists. Their level of supervision varies by state. Multiple state court decisions assert they cannot be sued personally when they are employed by another legal entity and are not legally required to follow the same standard of care as physicians.

the standard of care and their patient is harmed, regardless if they own their own practice or are employed by a hospital. This kind of liability is called *fiduciary responsibility*, where the responsible party—in this case, a physician—is legally required to act in the best interest of his or her beneficiary (patient).

Being a physician grants many privileges but not without corresponding responsibilities. If you don't want to take your medications, I can't abandon you. If you have a preexisting condition, I can't deny you care. If your surgery runs late, I must stay to finish it. If you need your appendix removed in the middle of the night, I must do the case. It doesn't matter how tired I am or how many hours I worked that day. If I don't want to treat you based on my personal beliefs, I must find another physician who will. As Harry Truman famously said in 1945, "The buck stops here."[50]

If a physician acts below the standard of care and causes harm, the patient can personally sue him or her because those actions violate fiduciary responsibility. Then if the lawsuit is successful and a physician doesn't have malpractice insurance or the malpractice coverage is not enough to cover the damages, the plaintiff can take the physician's life savings, house, and any other assets up to the awarded damages.

I find it strange other paid advice givers do not have the same level of responsibility. Economists, health gurus, financial advisors, political commentators, and fortune tellers are not legally required to give good advice. *Caveat emptor!* Buyer beware! These "professional" advice givers often give poor advice because they personally benefit from being lucky, but they don't face consequences for being wrong.

---

50 President Truman had a sign on his desk inscribed with "The buck stops here" on one side and "I'm from Missouri" on the other. A brief history of his sign can be found at trumanlibrary.gov.

In some circumstances, advice givers actually benefit from giving harmful advice. They have no incentive to give quality advice because they do not sustain a penalty for giving poor advice—in economics this is called moral hazard—where the party that does not pay the consequences of their actions incentivizes risky behavior to the detriment of the other party.

This chapter outlines the first way to better manage the synergy inherent in complex systems. *Skin in the game* means incurring personal liability as the result of an action. As a physician, this means every time I give medical advice to a patient or administer anesthesia, I stand to gain from a good outcome, but more importantly, I stand to lose from a poor outcome. Complex systems rely on both positive and negative feedback systems for stability. Skin in the game provides these two feedback loops: allowing safe doctors to continue practicing and culling dangerous ones from the herd.[51]

Anesthesiologists learn to manage complexity partly because we stand to lose everything if our patients suffer harm caused by our negligent actions. *Necessity is the mother of innovation.* As I discovered in medical school, doctors are highly incentivized, first culturally, then legally, to tell the truth and not be wrong.

§ PERSONAL PATIENTS §

Physicians learn skin in the game early in their training. During my intern year, I spent a month on the trauma surgery service. One of our patients was an elderly Hispanic gentleman who hadn't seen a doctor in decades. He had a slowly growing bulge in his right groin. Over 24 hours, he developed a high temperature,

---

51   In 2018, Nassim Taleb wrote a follow-up book to his *Incerto* series called *Skin in the Game: Hidden Asymmetries in Daily Life.* This chapter is an application of the concept.

elevated heart rate, and the bulge became exquisitely tender. He arrived in the emergency department for treatment.

He was admitted to the general surgery service for an incarcerated inguinal hernia, when a loop of bowel becomes stuck in a hole in the connective tissue surrounding the abdominal organs. If the loop of bowel becomes too stuck, the blood supply is cut off. Then the dying tissue releases bacteria and metabolic waste into the bloodstream. After some antibiotics and IV fluids, we took him to the operating room, fixed his hernia, and then planned his discharge from the hospital.

I was in charge of discharging him. He had a foley catheter in his bladder and an appointment to follow up with urology. He complained of pain from the catheter, a common grievance especially in men. He had no other signs of infection, so I decided not to give him antibiotics. I discharged him with close urology follow-up. I personally made the appointment. Two days later, I received a stern call from the junior surgical resident admitting patients from the emergency department. My patient was back. He had a urinary tract infection. The junior resident admitted him for IV antibiotics.

When my attending and I rounded on the surgery service, we stopped by his room last. My attending raised his eyebrows, looked at me, and said, "Go in and see him yourself; he is your personal patient." Then my attending walked away. I didn't want to face him and his family. He trusted me with his life and I failed him. Eventually, I took a deep breath, knocked, and entered the room. I will never forget the way his wife looked at me.

We both knew I was negligent. I should have prescribed the antibiotics to mitigate the risk of a urinary tract infection in a high-risk patient, and I chose not to do it. If his wife wasn't so diligent about his health, he might have stayed at home while the urinary tract infection worsened, and then he would have suffered additional complications such as kidney damage or surgical site infection. He could have been in the ICU on a ventilator and dialysis machine. I got lucky. The next day, he was discharged again, this time with a 14-day course of antibiotics.

The following year, I was scheduled to administer anesthesia for a young woman receiving spine surgery. The night before, I'd spent an hour scouring her chart to make sure I knew everything about her medical and surgical history. I noticed she had a recent urinalysis with bacteria in it. It was buried in an infrequently used section of the electronic medical record on the fourth page of a progress note.

Operating on patients with untreated bacterial infections can be disastrous, especially when hardware is implanted like in spine surgery. Bacteria can attach to the foreign material forming a biofilm resistant to antibiotics. Curing the infection usually requires additional surgeries and months of IV antibiotics.

Patients often have long-term pain and temporary or permanent disability. The surgeon and my attending were horrified because no one else had noticed the abnormal test until I mentioned it the morning of surgery. She was a young healthy woman in her 40s. Her surgery was postponed until the infection was properly treated.

Having the life of another person in your hands is always a personal matter between the patient and the physician. Everything else is superfluous. Physicians are indoctrinated to think in terms of radical accountability: taking ownership of your thoughts, actions, behavior, and results. Every lab result, vital sign, physical exam finding, patient complaint, and decision is ultimately your responsibility.

Medical school and residency are the places to learn this from attendings. Some teach with negative feedback, removing maladaptive thinking patterns. *Via negativa.* I sometimes think back to my month with Dr. Lucas and Dr. Ledgerwood. Years later, I can still feel Dr. Lucas's disappointment and hear Dr. Ledgerwood's yelling.

Our culture of radical accountability strongly incentivizes doctors to correctly triage uncertainty. Physician training is long, expensive, and complicated, but it works. High-quality care benefits both physicians and patients especially considering we will all be someone's patient one day.

In my primary care rotation of medical school, I saw an interesting example of radical accountability.

Miss A first contacted Dr. B's family practice in 2011 when she presented as a new patient with diabetes and high blood pressure. Dr. B helped manage Miss A's chronic diseases for the next two years. In 2013, when Miss A presented with new abdominal pain and swelling, Dr. B ordered a CT scan of her abdomen. It revealed a 5.5 cm mass initially diagnosed as a seroma, which is a collection of clear fluid usually found in the abdomen after surgery. However, Miss A had not had surgery. Subsequent surgical drainage revealed 40 cc of bloody fluid, initially diagnosed as a bruise.

Miss A came back to Dr. B in April 2014 when another CT scan revealed a 9 × 12.6 cm mass attached to her abdominal wall. Now, after a second surgical consultation, Miss A was diagnosed with a large hernia. As the mass grew larger, Miss A again turned to Dr. B who ordered yet another CT scan, which showed the mass was now 18 × 10 × 12 cm, about the size of a 2 L soda bottle.

Shortly thereafter, Miss A developed gastroenteritis, a self-resolving infection of the intestines. She was sent to the hospital by Dr. B for inpatient care. During her hospitalization, the mass was biopsied and diagnosed as cancer. Specialists recommended radiation first to shrink the tumor, followed by surgery to remove it. These plans were postponed due to an unforeseen complication: during another follow-up appointment with Dr. B, Miss A appeared short of breath. Miss A thought she was fine, refused to go to the hospital, and was adamant on picking up her grandson from his baseball game.

Dr. B convinced her to go to the hospital for a CT scan of her lungs. At the hospital, a massive blood clot was found in her lungs along with smaller blood clots in her legs. She spent ten days in the ICU and was eventually discharged on a blood thinner called warfarin.

Miss A proved very sensitive to warfarin. When her blood became dangerously thin, Dr. B recommended going to the emergency department for treatment. Warfarin overdose can cause internal bleeding. Additionally, Miss A could not start her cancer treatment if her blood was too thin. However, Miss A refused. She was tired of going to the hospital. Dr. B then found a health food store that carried the specific kind of vitamin K to partially reverse the warfarin. Now Miss A could start cancer treatment on time.

She completed six weeks of radiation followed by a seven-hour surgery. After she recovered in the hospital, she was admitted to a nursing home. Over the next three months, her surgical incision slowly healed.

I met Miss A in 2015, more than two years after she first presented to Dr. B with abdominal pain. Her incision had decreased in size from 90 cm (3 feet) to 20 cm (7.8 inches). She was ambulating with a walker and had a cheery disposition. Her journey was almost complete.

Radical accountability is taught in medical school and residency because physicians are also subject to moral hazard. The decisions they make are often life or death for their patients but not life and death for them. Physicians and their patients benefit most when doctors are socialized to make decisions as though every patient is a member of their family.

§ FIDUCIARY RESPONSIBILITY §

A culture of radical accountability is not enough. Every medical decision is viewed not only through a moral lens—*every patient should be treated like your family*—but also through a legal one.

The Hippocratic oath does not practice medicine; people do. At the individual level, medicine is an incomplete art practiced by imperfect humans. We live with limited perspective, limited experiences, and limited knowledge. We are prone to frustration, laziness, and taking shortcuts. Therefore, physicians are bound by medical malpractice laws to protect patients from physician fallibility.

First, let's define the legal definition of medical malpractice. Four things are required:

1. A fiduciary relationship existed. In this case, it is a formal doctor-patient relationship.
2. Deviation from standard of care.

3. The patient sustained harm.
4. The harm was caused by the deviation from standard of care.

Malpractice is *not* the same thing as a complication. For example, my PKD patient from Chapter 7 was not malpractice because I did not deviate from standard of care. In complex systems, some outcomes aren't predictable even when best practices are followed. Malpractice law (legal skin in the same) separates bad luck from bad decision makers.[52]

Malpractice is *not* the same thing as a correlation. For example, if I give a patient Tylenol for knee pain, then two hours later he suffers a heart attack, that doesn't mean the Tylenol caused the heart attack. Just because the Tylenol was given in close proximity to the heart attack doesn't mean the two are linked by causation. Correlation is not causation. Causation must be established for malpractice to exist.

Physician education focuses on the mechanisms of human physiology and medical treatments so they can navigate causation and correlation. Think back to Miss A: initially, her symptoms did not make sense in the context of her CT scan finding. Dr. B ordered the appropriate workup and follow-up until the correct diagnosis was found.

The ability to derive causation from a complicated clinical scenario is the calling card of a physician. That's also why physician education is long, complicated, and expensive. We don't spend more than a decade studying for our own enjoyment. We do it because it is necessary to successfully navigate complex domains.

---

52 "Bad luck events" are reported at conferences via case reports and poster presentations. Physician educational culture is built around explaining outcomes in the third layer of knowledge.

As an anesthesiologist, I need to know how normal physiology works, how abnormal physiology works, and how my anesthetic affects them both. Patients present with an infinite combination of symptoms, laboratory values, and imaging studies. Memorizing every pattern is impossible because an infinite number of patterns exist. Instead, physicians learn mechanisms so we can work from uncertainty to certainty. Ideally, our pursuit of certainty should be done in the safest way possible. Legal skin in the game incentivizes physicians to avoid unnecessary risks while deriving causation.

Holding anesthesiologists responsible for their choices is especially important because patients rarely choose their anesthesiologists and they cannot communicate their preferences while asleep. For perspective, patients can choose their surgeon or their primary care physician. They can take their time, get second opinions, and ask questions about every step in the treatment process. This does not really exist for anesthesiologists. Patients seem to be more scared of anesthesia than they are of surgery.

On the day of surgery, you show up and there I am! After a brief conversation, I take you to the operating room, push some drugs, and you are asleep. Suddenly, your life is in the hands of a stranger. Malpractice acts as an additional layer of safety for unconscious patients under anesthesia.[53]

§ ANESTHESIOLOGY, MALPRACTICE, AND PUBLISHING §

"Blaming anesthesia" is a sacred operating room tradition. Patient arrives late? Anesthesia's fault. Starbucks order was incorrect? Defi-

---

53   In the United States, medical malpractice law is far from perfect. In fact, some argue US malpractice laws incentivize doctors to practice lower quality, wasteful "defensive medicine." Excessive malpractice lawsuits probably don't improve quality of care versus fewer lawsuits. The *possibility* of lawsuits probably raises quality of care, but carrying out a clinical trial to measure that difference in quality (if any exists) would be unethical and unrealistic.

nitely anesthesia's fault. Global warming? Anesthesia was involved somehow. We accept this teasing with a sense of humor.

Under the tradition lies the subconscious recognition of an additional moral hazard. Surgeons manage post-operative complications even if the complications were caused by the anesthesiologist. In order to compensate for this unfair arrangement, surgeons will blame anesthesia for every problem in the operating room regardless of whose fault it was.

The additional moral hazard influences how anesthesiologists view liability. We are hyperfocused on documenting our medications, procedures, and reasoning such that none of our actions are linked to synergistic complications after surgery. The only objective record of our actions is our anesthesia record.

We craft our anesthetic as lawyers write a legal argument. We purposely document our actions in such a way to prove our actions made sense, were within the standard of care, and had greater potential benefits than harms. We don't want our actions to be associated with future post-operative complications for the good of the patient (and surgeon).

Our neurotic dedication to internal validity is a safety mechanism to make sure our patients receive high-quality care. We need to make sure every irregularity is explained when the case is over, so if any events occur in the future, the record protects us. If a complication occurs, we have already separated bad luck and malpractice (correlation and causation). Poor documentation makes us potentially liable for future complications. By focusing on future possible complications, anesthesiologists decrease the frequency of those complications.

Moral, legal, and cultural accountability forced anesthesiologists to become experts at thriving in uncertainty. Our outcomes continue to improve because we put skin in the game. We incentivize ourselves to *tell the truth and not be wrong.*

I applied the same concept to this book. When I started, I knew nothing about publishing, had limited writing experience, and didn't have any connections to the publishing world. Faced with the enormously complex task of publishing a book *during residency*, I fell back on my anesthesiology training. Perhaps I could leverage skin in the game?

Traditional publishing deals usually involve an author sending a book proposal to a publishing company who then pays the author an advance to write the book. The author functions as a screenwriter in that he or she sells the manuscript to the publishing company, and then the publishing company does the editing, cover design, and distribution. The author may not own legal or financial rights to the book or make the final decisions about the back-end publishing tasks. This model did not fit my values. I wanted to be radically accountable, so I was highly incentivized to *tell the truth and not be wrong.*

I chose to front the publishing costs myself instead of relying on an advance from a publishing company. Now I had financial skin in the game. Then I hired a publishing company called Scribe Media for a defined set of publishing tasks. That way, I have the final say in all decisions within the scope of our contract. Additionally, I own the intellectual property of the book. Now I have legal skin in the game. Then I shared my ideas with my family, friends, and colleagues. Now I have personal skin in the game.

This structure makes me maximally accountable for every part of the publication process, including writing the manuscript, editing, cover design, marketing, and distribution. If this book contains misinformation, grammatical errors, or faulty logic, I have no one to blame but myself. There is no diffusion of responsibility. As Harry Truman would say, "The buck stops here."

Typically, publishing companies will only publish books with large preexisting audiences because they earn most of their money through book sales. However, authors usually write books for nonmonetary reasons. None of my reasons for writing this book involved monetary gain, as outlined in the Introduction. An important idea may or may not be popular. Typically, authors have *soul in the game* and publishers have only financial skin in the game.

That means the writer and publisher may have different, even opposite, goals. For a publisher, it may be more profitable to change the content of a book at the expense of the author's purpose for writing the book. Opposite incentives can create an antagonistic relationship instead of a cooperative one.

In my arrangement, the publishing company is accountable to me instead of book sales. They get paid the same whether I sell ten or ten million copies. Instead of me focusing on writing a book for personal reasons while they try to maximize book sales, we are both focused on creating the highest quality book possible. We solved the moral hazard problem inherent in traditional publishing by aligning our values with our legal and financial structures.

Just as my publishing company is accountable to me, I am accountable to them. Before we chose to work together, they screened me for the internal validity of my idea, my insight into the applicability of those ideas, my expectations of the publishing process, and my work ethic. I made sure their expertise was consistent with my goals. I presented them with a detailed business plan before anyone signed a contract. Despite the fact I have the final say in all decisions, I take their feedback very seriously. Most of the time, I defer to their judgment because I am not an expert in book publishing; they are.

This book is written for the reasons outlined in the Introduction, but it is also a skin in the game experiment. I hypothesized I could apply skin in the game to the complex system of book publishing. I incentivized myself to *tell the truth and not be wrong* by making myself radically accountable for its content. I alone bear the consequences. You, the reader, will be the final judge of the result!

§ BETTER DECISIONS IN COMPLEX SYSTEMS §

Let's take a brief tour of how anesthesiologists put skin in the game, aka "buy into their complex system." First, we will examine time and then money.

The first way to make better decision makers is require a long buy-in of time. The more important the decision maker, the longer the buy-in.

To apply to medical school, an applicant must earn a four-year undergraduate degree, complete specific required science classes, and take the medical college entrance test (MCAT). Every medical school receives thousands of applications for about 150 spots per year. Medical schools take the best of the best: that means high test scores, high grades, volunteering, research, entrepreneurial ventures, and personal experiences are all factored into admissions criteria.

If you can get into medical school, you put even more skin in the game. In medical school, you work and study more than 80 hours per week for four years straight…and you don't get paid for it—in fact, *you pay for it.* The average medical student debt is about $240,000. During my third year of medical school, I explained this to a homeless man as I was walking to the hospital. He laughed at me as he walked away.[54]

After medical school, you cannot practice medicine independently. You must apply and be accepted by a residency program where you continue working and studying in a specific field. I chose anesthesiology. Resident physicians in the United States earn between $40,000 and $70,000 per year while the interest on their debt grows.[55]

In residency, you are formally tested every day by your patients and attendings. You take written and oral exams to make sure you know what you are supposed to know. Residency lasts between three and seven years. Finally after you pass your final board exams, you can start practicing independently.

Becoming a physician consumes at least 11 years of life. My training will consume a total of 16 years. This weeds out people who are "min/maxers," who want the most benefit for the least amount of effort. This kind of thinking is most compatible with the management of simple systems.

Although there is nothing inherently wrong with these people,

---

54 Medical school debt is not 100% necessary per se. However, high-quality basic science and clinical instruction costs money. If medical students want a high-quality education, they must realize there is no such thing as a free lunch. That being said, the rapid increase in medical school costs over the last 20 years is also not sustainable.

55 More information about the medical school admissions process can be found at students-residents.aamc.org. A comprehensive description is also included at the end of this book in Appendix II.

they are highly likely to permanently damage complex systems by making decisions based on a false simple system interpretation of reality. Complex system decision makers should be highly motivated people willing to dedicate an unreasonable amount of time to develop true expertise.

The second way to create better decision makers is by paying them a lot of money and making it easy for them to lose that money.

In the United States, physician compensation affords a level of financial security most people will never have. I would argue patients benefit from paying doctors well. Physician compensation gives them a financial incentive to protect their position—and the best way to do that is to practice responsibly.

The threat of losing their medical license or being sued is a very potent motivator for them to make the best decisions for their patients. A single act of negligence can end a physician's career or bankrupt him or her. The personal welfare of the decision maker must be tied to the performance of the complex system.

Put a different way, if physicians were not paid well and anyone could legally practice medicine, do you think quality of care would go up or down? A free market approach doesn't work because healthcare is a necessity, not an optional product or service. If you have a life-threatening illness you cannot choose to *not* purchase medical care. Market economies for non-essential products tend to function as simple systems. Complex systems, like medicine, play by more complicated rules.

Doctors make a considerable amount of money, certainly more than the average American. When you factor in undergraduate student loans, medical school debt, and lost income in medical school, the money might not be as good as you think. Additionally, doctors pay for malpractice insurance, licensing fees, and higher taxes as an employee or take on the additional financial responsibilities of running their own practice. If you are willing to work >80 hours per week for years on end *and* your priority is money, you will make more money in finance.

In summary, the elements for skin in the game are:

1. Large buy-in
2. Large reward at end
3. Easy to lose position or privilege

Think of skin in the game another way. If you have no penalties for saying something incorrect, you are essentially a fortune teller relying on confirmation bias to be "proven correct." A more appropriate setup for a fortune teller would be to award the fortune teller ten dollars for every correct prediction and make him or her pay ten dollars per incorrect prediction. That means they must be more than 50% accurate to be financially solvent. If this rule existed, how many fortune tellers would actually exist?[56]

People intuitively understand putting themselves at risk, but they oftentimes have poor insight into their own abilities. Skin in the game makes an individual think twice about whether he or she wants to link his or her destiny with his or her decisions. I find people love to talk about their opinions, but as soon as they

---

56 The first-person perspective (decision maker taking risks in the moment) and the third-person perspective (post-hoc observer with confirmation bias) are fundamentally different. Confirmation bias often develops in people who are not held responsible for their incorrect predictions. Those with the most confirmation bias seem to be the least likely to recognize their maladaptive thinking patterns. Psychologist Gary Klein described the first person model as "naturalistic decision making." More information can be found in his book *Sources of Power: How People Make Decisions.*

become liable for making a decision based on their opinions, they suddenly have fewer of them. Linking the well-being of the decision maker to his or her decisions increases the likelihood of those decisions being *true and not wrong*.

In the next chapter, we will consider why skin in the game incentivizes decision makers to focus their time and efforts on tail risks.

CHAPTER 11

Tail Risks

"The greatest victory is that which requires no battle."

—SUN TZU, *THE ART OF WAR*

"The best way to get out of trouble is to stay out of trouble."

—ANESTHESIOLOGIST PROVERB

Components of complex systems desire to be connected to one another. Like a bored puppy locked in a small apartment for an extended period of time, they will create chaos if left alone. *Nature abhors a vacuum.* Randomness lurks in the background waiting for a moment of weakness to synergistically propagate into a Black Swan. In the operating room, anesthesiologists tend to those synergistic components behind our blue curtain.

Remember the story of John from the Introduction? Initially, my untrained eye saw simplicity when the true reality was complexity. Just like the pediatric ICU, in the operating room, complex interactions are precisely controlled by anesthesiologists. John recovered uneventfully because the pediatric ICU physicians made many small upstream adjustments in his management so he wouldn't suffer complications.

Similarly, a good anesthetic is measured by *absence* of complications and *absence* of action. The best anesthetics look simple because the complex component is so well managed that it appears to be absent. Anesthesiologists view their job as dangerous because they spend the entire time blocking the propagation of random events into lethal complications. An outside observer sees routine. We see all of the Black Swans we neutralized just in time.

If objective reality has both simple and complex components, and the complex component is neutralized by the anesthesiologist, then only the simple component is seen by outside observers.

In the financial world, investment bankers call Black Swans *tail risks*. A tail risk is a form of investment risk where the chance of a price moving three standard deviations from the average is greater than that predicted by a normal curve. Remember those figures from Chapter 1? Like Black Swans, tail risks are the synergistic components of objective reality.

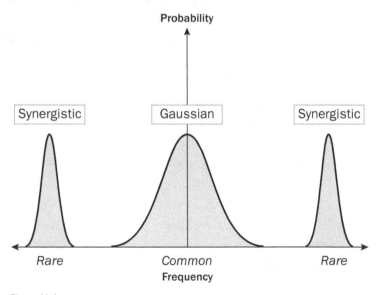

Figure 11-1

When those tail risks are absent, mathematical investing models based on the normal curve are valid. Success in the simple world of the normal distribution is logical and based on maximizing the success-to-failure ratio. Failure is encouraged as long as it means a net positive of lucky breaks.

However, success in complex systems is determined by the amount of time you survive. A single failure means game over. If you are killed by a Black Swan, you will never be able to harvest beneficial synergistic events later. Missing a beneficial event will not kill you. Missing a single tail risk event can, and will, kill you. Therefore, it benefits decision makers in complex systems to minimize tail risks.

Billion-dollar hedge funds like Melvin Capital exposed themselves to a tail risk in January 2021 when more than 100% of GameStop stock was "shorted." Shorting, aka short selling, is a financial contract where stock is borrowed and then immediately sold with a promise to buy it back at a future date. If the price is lower in the future, the investor keeps the difference (makes money). If the price is higher, the investor pays the difference (loses money).

Clever traders from an online community called Wall Street Bets on the social media site Reddit saw an opportunity. They aggressively bought the stock, driving up its price. This triggered short sellers to close their positions (buy back the stock) to prevent future losses, which then triggered more purchasing of the stock by r/wallstreetbets traders. This event is known as a short squeeze where limited supply of shorted stock and high demand causes a rapid increase in stock price. The stock price increased from $15 in December 2020 to a peak of $347 per share on January 27, 2021.

By the end of January 2021, short sellers lost an estimated $70 billion. Melvin Capital alone lost about $6 billion, approximately

50% of its value. If Robinhood, a stock trading app used by many r/wallstreetbets traders, hadn't halted trading of GameStop stock, hedge funds like Melvin Capital could have gone bankrupt. GameStop stock remains remarkably volatile—after decreasing to $40 per share in February 2021, it rose again to $240 per share in March 2021. The saga is far from over.[57]

Anesthesiologists are solely focused on these tail risks because a failure means their patient is dead. There are no loans, bailouts, or second chances in the operating room. Our methods developed with no margin for error. We thrive in our highly synergistic environment because the prevention of tail risks is the primary factor in our decision making.

§ FAT-TAILED DISTRIBUTIONS §

Tail Risks transform a normal curve into a fat-tailed distribution. A fat-tailed distribution appears below. Common events occur in the middle. Rarer events occur as you go left and right.

---

57 In the last days of January 2021, Robinhood prevented traders from buying more GameStop stock. The decision was controversial. Robinhood's CEO, Vlad Tenev, stated he halted trading because his company didn't have the collateral to cover the massive transfers of capital. Others saw it as market manipulation. More information about this event can be located in *The New York Times*, *The Wall Street Journal*, *Forbes*, and Reddit.

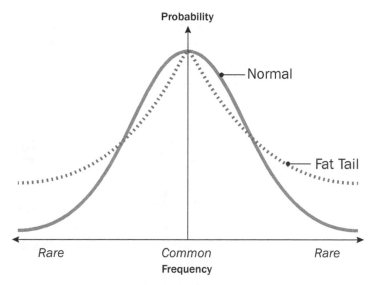

Figure 11-2

"Fat tails" are the addition of Black Swans to the normal distribution.

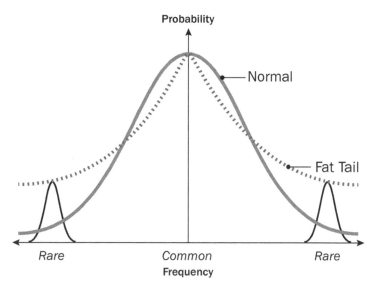

Figure 11-3

Tail Risks in finance are very different from tail risks in anesthesiology, but the concept is the same. Both are rare unpredictable events that cause large asymmetric fluctuations in a complex system. In finance, that means prices move more than three standard deviations than predicted. In anesthesiology, that means life-threatening events such as bradycardia, hypoxia, and hypotension. In finance, the events cause bankruptcy; in anesthesiology, they cause patient death.

Despite the fact that tail risks can be markedly different, strategies used by anesthesiologists might be widely applicable across different disciplines. If synergy is caused by complexity, lowering the complexity of any system will decrease its synergy. If synergy is decreased, the complex component of the distribution will shrink.

Anesthesiologists decrease synergy so much that 99% of the time, anesthesiology appears to have no synergy at all; it looks like a simple system. Anesthesiologists do this in two ways: disassociating components from one other and obtaining a comprehensive knowledge of the system components.

§ LINKAGE §

Tail Risks, synergy, and Black Swans are created when a single choice is linked to additional hidden decisions. Think of COVID-19. We might be in contact with only five people, but if those five people are in contact with five additional people and those 25 people have five contacts each, you are actually sharing germs with more than 100 people...without even knowing it. A single choice to be around five new people actually contains more than 100 hidden synergistic social contacts.

Linkage can also be observed in the United States political system.

Because there are only two parties, a voter who feels very strongly for or against a certain issue—such as criminal justice reform—might have to prioritize that belief over another belief they feel less strongly about. Their vote has many synergistically linked choices, including tax reform, immigration policy, and healthcare.

Voters might find themselves voting against some (or many) of their own interests in order to vote for a single issue. Cause and effect in these kinds of systems is difficult to measure because there is a significant degree of synergistic linkage. The consequences of a single choice are much greater than the choice alone. The solution might be a multiparty system. If a greater diversity of parties were present, voters could choose the specific party that best represents their true preferences.[58]

We see linkage in anesthesiology when we give drugs with side effects. One example is succinylcholine, a muscle relaxant used to paralyze a patient before intubation. In addition to its muscle relaxant properties, it has many undesirable side effects, including dangerous drops in heart rate, jaw spasms, cardiac arrest, and a hypermetabolic state called malignant hyperthermia. These are all synergistically linked to its primary usage.

When I choose succinylcholine, I choose its side effects too. Similarly, if I choose the Democratic Party for their ideas about education, I also must choose their ideas about immigration. I might not like their ideas about immigration, but I must accept them if I want their ideas about education.

Anesthesiologists prefer drugs that have one function, act quickly, are metabolized quickly, and have no secondary metabolites. We

---

58   I leave the design of government up to more qualified individuals than myself. I'm presenting multiple applications of a single idea in order to establish a conceptual pattern.

give as few drugs as possible to decrease the chance of unforeseen synergistic side effects. When manipulating an airway, such as inserting a breathing tube, we do it with as few actions as possible. The cords to our monitors (blood pressure, EKG, pulse oximetry, etc.) are untangled and given slack so if one is pulled out, the others are unaffected. Our breathing circuit and IV are separated from the monitor cords so they can also move independently. Even our anesthesia machine is designed so all the systems fail independently—meaning a single error in one part of the machine will not propagate into a massive system failure.

Error propagation cannot occur if the first mistake is not connected to other parts of the system. If one monitor is accidentally pulled off, none of the others will be affected. If my anesthesia machine fails, I can quickly diagnose and then fix the problem. If I see a complication, I can figure it out faster if I use the fewest and simplest drugs. Anesthesiologists even design their mistakes to be easily recognized and quickly solved.

During my first month of anesthesiology training, I was anesthetizing a craniotomy patient for brain tumor resection. After the patient was induced and intubated, a Mayfield device was attached to the patient's head. The Mayfield acts as a clamp, holding the head still during brain surgery. The pins are very sharp and very stimulating, so anesthesiologists usually give medications to prevent dangerous increases in heart rate and blood pressure. If untreated, the heart rate can increase to the 150s and blood pressure to 250 mmHg (normal systolic blood pressure is 120 mmHg). Pathologically high blood pressure and heart rates can cause life-threatening complications.

I prepared by lining up all of my drugs on my anesthesia cart. I reached for esmolol, a drug that lowers heart rate and blood pressure. I gave 50 mg, a safe and effective dose for my patient. Then I looked at the syringe in disbelief. Instead of esmolol, I gave ephedrine, a medication that raises both blood pressure and heart rate. Additionally, I gave five times the usual dose!

Now I had seconds to fix the problem. I quickly gave a hefty dose of propofol and *real* esmolol to counteract the pinning and ephedrine. As the medications dripped into my patient's veins, the Mayfield pins pierced his skin and penetrated his skull. His blood pressure and heart rate didn't move. However, MY blood pressure and heart rate skyrocketed! My mistake could have given my patient a stroke.

I knew my next mistake could be more serious and I may not be able to rescue myself in the future. So I created a system of drawing up and storing drugs so I couldn't make another drug error. I developed my own habits for labeling uppers and downers (medications that raise and lower the blood pressure).

I decreased the number of drugs I drew up in advance. I now only keep the drugs I'm highly likely to use in view; all others are kept out of sight. Before drawing up a drug, I hold the glass vial in front of my face, then I draw it up into a syringe. Before giving the drug, I hold the syringe in front of my face. After that one mistake, I have given tens of thousands of drugs without a single error.

By isolating the individual components of the complex system, I could decrease its synergy and therefore decrease synergistic complications. Anesthesiologists tend to be neurotic, compulsive organizers because they intuitively understand how linkage leads to synergistic complications. We understand success is not measured by "cost-benefit efficiency"; it is measured by avoiding Black Swans.

§ PREDICTING THE UNPREDICTABLE §

After the parts of a complex system are separated into individual components, the second part of tail risk prevention is acquiring a comprehensive knowledge of those components. Because Black Swans are by definition random, a broad base of knowledge increases the chances of already knowing the answer to an unpredictable problem.[59]

Reality does not neatly divide itself into medical specialties. Physicians all share the same basic education because a patient can have any disease at any time. The presentation of disease can be very variable, from obvious symptoms found on WebMD, unexpected symptoms in an academic journal, to no symptoms at all. Physicians must understand the context of every piece of clinical information. The common education we all share enables us to know what we know, know what we don't know, ask the right questions, and communicate effectively.

I saw one of my attendings do exactly this on my emergency medicine month of intern year. We had a healthy 65-year-old woman who came into the emergency department for acid reflux. She had no other medical problems. She had symptoms of acid reflux for years well controlled with an over-the-counter medication. Two days ago, she simply ran out of medication because she forgot to refill it before visiting her family in Los Angeles.

She had a normal EKG, a measurement of the electrical activity of the heart. She was insistent she go home so she could get back to her family party. She was given acid reflux medication and was already feeling better. She already had labs drawn, which were all normal. Considering we had a stack of untouched charts and a

---

59 A comprehensive discussion in favor of general education prior to specialization can be found in *Range: Why Generalists Triumph in a Specialized World* by David Epstein.

full waiting room, we could have sent her home. I already had two charts in my hands. But my attending spent 15 minutes, which is an eternity in an emergency room, convincing her to stay.

She wanted a troponin test just to make sure this wasn't a heart attack. Troponin is a cardiac muscle protein. High levels in the blood usually mean heart damage indicative of a heart attack. My attending sighed and said, "I would rather have a negative Yelp review than miss a heart attack, especially in a healthy 65-year-old woman with an active social life, ten grandkids, and vacation planned for next month."

A heart attack without EKG changes would be extremely unlikely, especially in a healthy patient. Furthermore, our patient got better after we gave her heartburn medication. We did everything right. At the time, I thought the additional test was a waste of time and money.

When the test came back positive, my jaw dropped. She was having a heart attack in front of my eyes. And I would have sent her home without treatment! My attending looked me straight in the eyes and said:

> I am constantly given different productivity standards and treatment algorithms. Administrators say the emergency department is wasteful. I would like those people to tell our patient her troponin test was wasteful. If she went to an urgent care, she would have been given acid reflux medication, sent home, then died in her sleep. I want you to remember your first priority is not to your ego, a paycheck, or an administrator. Your only priority is the patient in front of you.

I called the cardiology fellow, who arrived 15 minutes later, and then transported her to the cardiac catheterization lab. That night, he and his attending placed two stents in her right coronary artery.

My attending had abundant knowledge about the presentations, diagnosis, treatment, and outcomes of cardiovascular disease in women even though she wasn't a cardiologist. The American Heart Association didn't make its first consensus statement on acute myocardial infarction in women until 2016, nine years after my attending finished residency. Her broad knowledge of cardiovascular risk factors in women saved the life of our patient.[60]

Medical education is highly standardized to make sure every graduating physician understands the mechanisms of disease. The first two years we learn anatomy, histology, physiology, biochemistry, pharmacology, immunology, and pathophysiology in order to understand disease at its most basic level. That knowledge is integrated in third-year rotations of family medicine, internal medicine, surgery, pediatrics, obstetrics, gynecology, psychiatry, and neurology. Fourth-year rotations are electives for furthering clinical education in a specific area.

Then every newly minted physician must complete an intern year to fortify their clinical judgment under the watchful eye of attending physicians. Only after this common education do physicians specialize. For anesthesiology, we spend an additional three years in residency applying our broad education in the operating room. We need to isolate every component of the operating room complex system, learn everything about the individual parts, then practice recombining the individual elements in thousands of unique clinical scenarios.

---

60 The guidelines are "Acute Myocardial Infarction in Women: A Scientific Statement from the American Heart Association," by Dr. Laxmi S. Mehta published in *Circulation* in 2016.

Anesthesiologists take care of a wide range of patients: both children and the elderly, both healthy and sick, both scheduled cases and emergencies. On any given day, my first patient could be a healthy five-year old who needs his tonsils removed, the next could be a young woman who needs a breast cancer operation, then my third could be a critically ill elderly man with a perforated colon who needs emergency bowel surgery. My broad education allows me to understand how diffcrent synergistic factors organize into Black Swans so I can avoid the tail risks of unique situations I have never seen before.

In my fourth year of residency, I was called to the floor to intubate a woman in her 80s with aortic stenosis and chronic kidney disease on dialysis. Her heart rate was 140 beats per minute in an abnormal rhythm called atrial fibrillation. Blood pressure was dangerously low at 70/40 mmHg. Her respiratory rate was 40 per minute and she was dramatically short of breath. In this situation, I had about 15 seconds to make a decision only knowing two facts about her. The nurses and respiratory therapists demanded I intubate her or treat her new erratic heart rhythm.

Instead, I ordered IV fluids and magnesium. At first, everyone in the room was confused, but within 15 minutes, her vital signs returned to normal. We calmly wheeled her to the ICU for the night where her cardiac arrythmia resolved within the hour. She was transferred to the floor the following morning. Intubation or anti-arrhythmic medications probably would have killed her.

I correctly predicted all of her problems stemmed from recent dialysis exacerbated by her diseased heart valve. The dialysis removed too much fluid, so I replaced it. The magnesium stabilized her heart so her arrythmia wouldn't get worse. Thanks to my broad education, I correctly predicted her underlying problem and then treated it safely, quickly, and effectively, despite having no prior knowledge of her condition and not seeing this combination of diseases before. She was discharged from the hospital three days later without further complications.

The broader my knowledge, the more likely I will recognize synergistic propagation before Black Swans occur. My nephrology rotation in medical school bolsters my ability to understand the physiology and treatment of chronic kidney disease. My cardiac anesthesiology experience gave me expertise in valvular heart disease. My diverse ICU experiences taught me how to manage emergencies of every organ system. The broad education of medical school and residency gives me the ability to recognize potential tail risks, then create a plan to decrease synergy before a Black Swan occurs.

§ DECREASING THE CHANCE OF TAIL RISKS §

In summary, the following are two strategies to decrease synergy in complex systems to better manage tail risks:

- Separate the parts of the complex system into independent simple systems. Learn their histories, mechanisms of action, structure, and functions.
- Understand how simple systems interact to become complex systems. Complex systems exhibit Black Swans, synergy, the time paradoxes, propagation, and iatrogenesis.

Theories can predict the probability of an event happening, but they can't tell a decision maker how to proceed in a unique situation. Statistical models often break down in individual situations because a unique situation cannot be a percentage of an outcome. A person cannot have 10% of a heart attack. They either have a heart attack or they don't. In high-synergy situations, statistics become even less useful because every situation is infinitely unique.

When I entered residency four years ago, I was shocked at the infinite uniqueness of every patient. Suddenly, I had to think through every situation in terms of uncertainty and consequences rather than the textbook answer. In medical school, we say, "Patients don't read textbooks." Turns out I had to read the textbooks instead.

A disconnect will always exist between mathematical efficiency and catching Black Swans. Swan hunting is inefficient in the short term but efficient in the long term. The same concept applies to medical education. Teaching medical students and residents is tedious, frustrating, and expensive. In the long term, the investment pays for itself many times over because well-trained doctors are the only people who can sort through the complexity of disease. The final chapter will conclude our Swan hunt by introducing the concept of convexity.

CHAPTER 12

Convexity

"We want perfection without practice. Yet everyone is harmed if no one is trained for the future."

—Dr. Atul Gawande

"Honesty is a very expensive gift. Do not expect it from cheap people."

—Warren Buffett

When I was in my third year of medical school, I started CrossFit. CrossFit is part fitness program, part dance party, and part cult. It is a mixture of bodyweight movements, Olympic weightlifting, and gymnastics performed at high intensity. When I learned the barbell and gymnastics movements for the first time, my coaches were very strict about proper technique. They would say, "Slow is smooth, and smooth is fast." What they meant was, "Focusing on the proper form rather than constantly trying to lift the heaviest weight possible will grant sustainable gains over time."

Athletes improve by focusing on the fundamentals, accepting criticism, and working on their weaknesses. There is no cheating the process. I had to set my ego aside even when I saw girls lift more weight than me or beat me in workouts. It took me about a year to develop the proper wrist, shoulder, spine, hip, and ankle flexibility to do the basic movements correctly. Within two years, I could snatch my body weight, clean and jerk 1.5x my body weight, and back squat 2x my body weight. I also learned muscle-ups, one-legged squats, and how to walk on my hands.

At the same time, I saw some of my friends hurt themselves because they wanted to lift heavy but lacked the discipline to learn the fundamentals. They insisted they didn't need to stretch, that structured weightlifting programs were too boring, and that accessory exercises were unnecessary. One by one, they injured themselves.

Why do CrossFitters generally fall into two categories—those who progress too fast and injure themselves and those who slowly continue improving over time? Nassim Taleb would point to a phenomenon he calls convexity, which describes how a system responds to increasing complexity. CrossFit exposes the body to randomly assorted challenges of strength, power, and endurance. Athletes who can adapt to the random challenges will become stronger. Those who cannot adapt end up injured.[61]

As complexity increases, some systems display a lag time followed by slow, unlimited progress (positive convexity), and some display initial rapid progress followed by accelerating deterioration until they ultimately fail (negative convexity). I experienced positive convexity and improved over time with heavier weights and more complex movements because I heavily invested in mastering the fundamentals.

---

61   Convexity is mentioned in Nassim Taleb's *Antifragile: Things that Gain from Disorder*, Chapter 18.

Some of my friends without those fundamentals experienced negative convexity and injured themselves instead. To have positive convexity, you must be willing to take limited short-term penalties for unlimited long-term benefits. Unfortunately, some people choose to pursue limited short-term benefits at the expense of unlimited long-term penalties.

Systems with negative convexity will suffer from increasing complexity, such as my CrossFit friends who injured themselves. On the other hand, systems set up with positive convexity thrive under complexity and grow stronger over time. The two are shown graphically below.

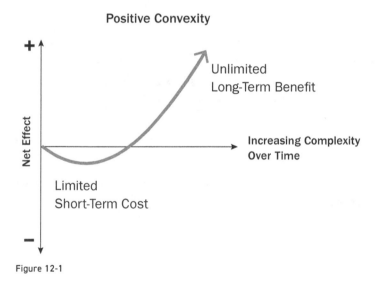

Figure 12-1

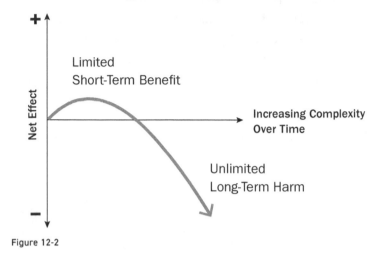

Negative Convexity

Limited
Short-Term Benefit

Increasing Complexity
Over Time

Net Effect

Unlimited
Long-Term Harm

Figure 12-2

The principles of positive convexity are probably not limited to CrossFit. They seem to be common across almost all disciplines, including medicine. Comprehensive knowledge, constructive criticism, and focus on the fundamentals leads to expertise over time.

The question is whether you are playing the short game or the long game. In complex systems, *failure is self-inflicted and excellence is self-bestowed.* In this final chapter, you will understand why anesthesiologists exhibit positive convexity

§ PHYSICIAN CONVEXITY §

Physician training wasn't always rigorous and standardized. In the late 1800s, there was a hodgepodge of medical practitioners in the United States. The public could not tell a real doctor from a quack. The word *quack* is a shortened version of the Dutch word *kwaksalver*, meaning "a hawker of medical salve." The word became synonymous with people who claimed to be medical experts without the knowledge or experience to back it up (false experts).

In 1910, the Carnegie Foundation commissioned a well-known American educator named Abraham Flexner to create a comprehensive summary of medical education in the United States and Canada. He visited all 155 medical schools and then wrote a book-length report called the *Flexner Report*.[62]

His main recommendations were:

1. Reduce the number of poor quality medical schools to decrease the number of poor quality practitioners.
2. Increase and standardize prerequisites for medical training especially in the basic sciences.
3. Train physicians in a scientific manner and engage in scientific research.
4. Medical students should receive hands-on instruction in hospitals by dedicated faculty.
5. Increase state regulation of medical licensure to make sure every medical practitioner meets minimum standards.

In 1904, there were 160 doctorate-granting medical schools. By 1935, there were only 60. Unproven and harmful medical practices, such as homeopathy, phrenology, and electrotherapy, were removed in favor of rigorous educational standards, the scientific method, and hands-on experience. Today, there are 155 MD-granting institutions and 36 DO-granting institutions, a total of 191 medical schools. The surviving DO schools today

---

62   Pages 9–173 of the *Flexner Report* contain the bulk of Flexner's recommendations. An academic summary is "Commentary: Understanding the Flexner Report" by Dr. Kenneth Ludmerer published in *Academic Medicine* in 2010.

abide by the same rigorous medical education standards as MD schools.[63]

Later in the 1900s, physician education became heavily regulated to ensure quality. The Liaison Committee on Medical Education (LCME) was founded in 1942 to make sure medical schools were teaching medical students what they needed to learn. The Liaison Committee for Graduate Medical Education (LCGME) was founded in 1972 and then expanded in 1981 to the Accreditation Council for Graduate Medical Education (ACGME) to make sure physician residency and fellowship programs were teaching new doctors how to practice medicine appropriately. State licensing boards were created as clearinghouses to make sure practicing physicians met educational standards. In less than a hundred years, quackery transformed into modern medicine.[64]

As I've detailed throughout this book, physicians can correctly sort objective reality into simple and complex systems, identify the three layers of knowledge, separate Systems 1 and 2, manage Black Swans, outmaneuver the time paradoxes, control propagation, and avoid iatrogenesis. But we can only do this after a long gestation period.

Our education grants us positive convexity, and anesthesiology is no exception to this rule. For the last 80 years, anesthesiologists systemically hunted Black Swans to the brink of extinction. We thrive in uncertainty because we set ourselves up to do so. *Structure determines function.*

---

63 In 2021, the degrees are essentially equivalent. MD stands for Doctor of Medicine; DO stands for Doctor of Osteopathic Medicine. As of July 2020, all residency programs abide by the same ACGME standards written by MDs. This means all MDs and DOs are trained to the same standard in residency.

64 More information about the LCME and ACGME can be found on their websites: acgme.org and lcme.org.

Below is a chart describing physician convexity.

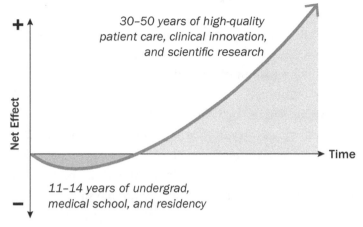

Figure 12-3

My education has been a decade-long physical and psychological war of attrition. I have passed five board exams, completed at least 50,000 multiple-choice questions, and spent approximately 14,000 hours actively participating in clinical decision making. I am finally at the inflection point of the convexity graph—where both my patients and I see the dividends of our shared investment.

§ CAN DOCTORS BE REPLACED? §

Training doctors is expensive, it takes a long time, and it can't happen everywhere. Medical schools and residency programs are bound by very strict standards set by the LCME and ACGME in order to make sure the American public has access to high-quality physicians. To maximize the number of patients treated by physicians, mid-level providers were invented to offset routine clinical work. "Mid-levels" have more education than medical assistants or nurses but still much less than physicians. A mid-level provider and a physician are analogous to a paralegal and a lawyer, veterinary technician and a veterinarian, or flight attendant and pilot.

They are best suited for narrow tasks carried out under the supervision of a physician. Examples include a primary care NP working longitudinally with uncontrolled diabetic patients or a PA discharging routine patients from the hospital while an orthopaedic surgeon is operating. They do not understand medicine like physicians do because they do not have our rigorous, standardized education. The term *mid-level* objectively describes their level of education: "in the middle." They are sometimes known as advanced practice providers (APPs) or nonphysician providers (NPPs). For the rest of this chapter, they will be referred to as NPPs.

Below is a summary of the three main types of NPPs.

- Physician assistant (PA): 26 months, master's degree, assists physicians in a variety of clinical areas, including the emergency department, outpatient clinics, and in the operating room. Most standardized.
- Nurse anesthetist (CRNA): 25–50 months, master's degree, assists anesthesiologists in the operating room monitoring patients during surgical procedures. They are an ICU nurse for the operating room.
- Nurse practitioner (NP): 12–24 months, partially to fully online degree, often done part time while working as a nurse, no quality control, optional clinical training. Least standardized.

Below is an infographic comparing supervised clinical training hours of NPPs and physicians. Previous experience in a related field is not included because carrying out tasks is different from understanding why the task needs to be done. Additionally, practicing without expert feedback is not considered high-quality training.[65]

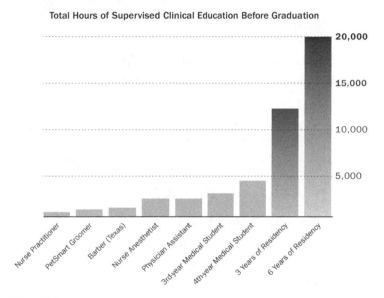

Total Hours of Supervised Clinical Education Before Graduation

Figure 12-4

NPPs represent a short-term solution to the rising demand for healthcare services. Teaching and education takes up a lot of time and resources that could be spent building a new cancer center

---

65   PA: aapa.org/wp-content/uploads/2016/12/Issue_Brief_PA_Education.pdf

CRNA: Council on Accreditation of Nurse Anesthesia Educational Programs. Standards for accreditation of nurse anesthesia educational programs. Approved 2004, revised June 2016.

Texas Barber: tdlr.texas.gov/barbers/barberfaq.htm#1500-to-1000

PetSmart Groomer: services.petsmart.com/grooming

NP: "Family Nurse Practitioner Clinical Requirements: Is the Best Recommendation 500 Hours?" by Christell Bray, published in the *Journal of the American Academy of Nurse Practitioners* in 2009.

or a new outpatient surgery building to keep up with patient demand. Hospitals could become more efficient by hiring NPPs to assist the physicians they already had. They also represented a short-term solution to the physician shortage. NPPs are easier and cheaper to train because their educational standards are lower.

NPPs hail themselves as the future of healthcare. As of January 2021, 28 state legislatures have granted independent practice privileges to NPs without educational standards or legal oversight. PAs and CRNAs are also lobbying state governments for independent practice privileges despite lacking the knowledge, metacognition, and experience to do so safely.

There is not a single study showing NPPs can safely make independent clinical decisions. All studies are so poorly designed that their results are meaningless, inconclusive, or show NPPs provide worse quality of care at the same or higher cost. Studies *do* show patient outcomes are similar with physicians alone or physicians with supervised NPPs.[66]

To make matters more confusing, NPP academic administrators created nonclinical doctorate degrees. CRNAs created doctorates of nurse anesthesia practice (DNAP), PAs created doctorates of medical science (DMSc), and NPs created doctorates of nursing practice (DNP).

None of them are equivalent to an MD or DO, which is a true

---

66 A comprehensive list of studies about independent NPPs is included in the book *Patients at Risk: The Rise of the Nurse Practitioner and Physician Assistant in Healthcare* by Dr. Rebekah Bernard and Dr. Niran Al-Agba. As of 2021, no study has shown independent NPPs are equivalent to physicians. Studies have shown independent NPPs obtain more consults, prescribe more opiates, do not improve rural access to healthcare, and do not decrease healthcare expenditures compared to physician-led care. Current data suggests independent NPPs might provide worse care at an equivalent or higher cost. The findings are consistent with the significant differences in training.

doctorate-level education for the diagnosis and treatment of disease. This difference can be very confusing in a clinical setting if an NPP has a nonclinical "doctorate" but is not a physician. These new "doctorates" raise the question of quackery. Are they practicing medicine independently? If so, why are they practicing medicine without a medical education or medical license?

Physicians and NPPs both have their roles in high-quality patient care. They create value in different ways at different times for different reasons. Physicians create value by directing diagnosis and treatment. NPPs do not have this ability because they do not have the rigorous education of medical school and residency. It is not a question of personal value; it is a question of high-quality training.

NPPs, an increasingly corporatized healthcare structure, and rising demand for healthcare services has created a powerful politico-economic engine for negative convexity. An independent NPP is like a CrossFitter with poor form. The outcome is iatrogenic injury.

Like a weightlifter who tries to lift heavy weight without proper technique, NPPs cause permanent harm when they are given the complex responsibilities of a physician. They lack the ability to function in complex domains because they lack high-quality physician training.

Until the 1990s, there was a relative balance of physicians and NPPs. However, the Balanced Budget Act of 1997, a federal law limiting Medicare spending, prevented future increases in federal funds for residency programs. Many people, including physicians, don't realize the federal government subsidizes physician residency training. During the last 24 years, no additional public money has become available to fund these programs despite an exponential increase in healthcare demand and a 24% increase in medical student enrollment.[67] The physician shortage has become a physician crisis.

At the same time, NPP training has proliferated. The Bureau of Labor Statistics projects NPPs to grow more than four times faster than physicians.[68] For perspective, the number of NPs doubled between 2010 and 2017 from 91,000 to 190,000. In 2016, there was fewer than one NP per five physicians. In 2030, there will be two NPs per five physicians.[69]

The rapid proliferation of NPPs makes training doctors more difficult. If NPPs are taking away clinical opportunities from medical students and residents, how can we train more doctors? The solution for a physician shortage is more physicians, not more NPPs. The physician shortage is propagated by overconfident NPPs lobbying state governments for independence practice and doctors remaining silent about their lack of residency spots.

In simple systems, errors tend to be fixed as they occur because they are knowable. In complex systems, errors tend to propagate outside of our perception until they organize into catastrophic Black Swans. Negative convexity is a formidable force of destruction. Without intervention, physician education may sustain irreversible damage. There may come a point in the future when patients no longer have access to physicians.

---

67 aamc.org/media/49911/download.

68 bls.gov, Occupational Outlook Handbook.

69 An accessible summary of NP growth can be found in the journal *Health Affairs*. The article is titled "Implications of the Rapid Growth of the Nurse Practitioner Workforce in the US" by David Auerbach, published in 2020.

§ NEGATIVE CONVEXITY...EVERYWHERE §

Negative convexity is also seen in our economics, where we prioritize limited short-term gains in exchange for unlimited future harms. The short-term financial success of deregulation had hidden future liabilities now being paid by the millennial generation as high-interest educational debt, rising housing costs, unsustainable cost of living, and low incomes.

In the United States, millennials (born 1981–1996) currently make up the largest population demographic but own only 3.2% of total assets. At the same age, baby boomers (born 1946–1964) owned 21%. As complexity increases over time, our economic convexity appears to be negative. Future generations are doing worse instead of better.[70]

Negative convexity can be observed in almost every aspect of our failing society: banks "too big to fail" that easily go bankrupt, private ownership of public resources, and the 2020 United States COVID-19 response. We are now seeing the unlimited harms, including catastrophic Black Swans, caused by a few decades of negative convexity. Limited, short-term benefits are now overshadowed by unlimited future harms, including Black Swans, fracturing the infrastructure of our political, social, and economic institutions.

Negative convexity occurs when decision makers treat reality as a simple system: they aim for short-term efficiency rather than long-term viability. Simple decision makers tend to have no skin in the game, don't understand the unique tail risks of their systems, and don't factor synergistic complications into their decisions. Short-term "efficiencies" eventually cause inevitable collapse.

---

70 In 2019, Christopher Ingraham published an excellent graphic in *The Washington Post*. The article's title is "The Staggering Millennial Wealth Deficit, in One Chart."

§ POSITIVE CONVEXITY §

In complex systems, success is measured in longevity. As time passes, the benefits of learning compound exponentially while the cost of learning decreases. Eventually, the benefits of expertise exceeds the cost of learning, and positive convexity occurs.

Anesthesiologists accept limited short-term losses in exchange for avoiding catastrophic Black Swans just as a CrossFit athlete (should) accept slower progress in exchange for avoiding injury. A single catastrophic injury can cause permanent physical disability, just as a single error can cause patient death. Complex systems are mastered by preventing Black Swans, not by maximizing growth.

Mastery requires a commitment to learning. True learning requires unpleasantness, frustration, and sadness as your psychology and nervous system slowly change to perceive true complexity rather than false simplicity. It also means finding out you might know less than you think and are wrong more often than you would like. Progress is not always obvious or measurable. Learning takes more time than you think for fewer results than you think you deserve.

Positive convexity means investing time and money studying uncertainty, and focusing on what is unknown rather than what is known. Anesthesiology became safer as patients became more complicated because anesthesiologists are willing to suffer for 12 years to truly master the complex system of anesthesiology. Our educational standards compounded over decades to yield unprecedented results. The standard in anesthesiology is perfection. This book has outlined what we learn, how we learn it, and how experience validates our knowledge and metacognition in objective reality.

As I look back on my medical education and forward to my future,

I realize the study of uncertainty is not a task to be completed. It is a tradition meant to be passed down. In fact, the word *doctor* is based on the Latin word *docere*, meaning "to teach." I hope you have learned something useful from this book.

I spent my entire adult life enduring constant physical exhaustion, sustaining continuous psychological stress, and balancing on a tightrope between life and death. I never knew when I would leave the hospital. Turns out I was in the right place the whole time.

And I have no regrets.

Conclusion

"We don't rise to the level of our expectations; we fall to the level of our training."

—Archilochus, Greek poet

"We must all suffer from one of two pains in life: the pain of discipline or the pain of regret."

—Jim Rohn

Between my first and second years of medical school, I observed medical uncertainty for the first time while working on a blood clotting assay. After congenital heart surgery, some patients require the implantation of an artificial shunt to redirect blood flow around the heart. Blood clots tend to form inside the shunt, so aspirin, a blood thinner, is given to babies after surgery to prevent the blood clots. My task was to identify the differences in blood clotting using an experimental clotting assay before and after giving aspirin to the babies.

Every day for a month straight, I rounded with the pediatric ICU team, collected blood samples, then tested them in an experimental clotting assay. In order to make sure the blood didn't clot before I could run my experiments, I would take it directly from the hospital to my laboratory. I couldn't afford a single mistake—I needed to run more than 20 assays with only 4 ml of blood. I made detailed checklists to make sure I followed all of the protocols exactly. I was too scared to even go to the bathroom because that would mean letting the blood out of my sight.

One day, after finishing tests on the blood of my fifth patient, I walked west on Canfield Street from my laboratory in the Elliman Building to La Palma, a popular Mediterranean restaurant frequented by Wayne State medical students. As I ate my chicken shawarma pita, I watched stoplights change at the intersection of Canfield and Brush Street. Eventually, I lost myself in thought.

That morning, after looking at my data, I noticed a pattern: some babies' blood responded to the aspirin and some didn't. For a brief moment, I realized I might know something no one else in the world knew. Was one group more susceptible to blood clots than the other?

If I was the pediatric ICU physician, would I trust this test to guide clinical decision making? What would I do if one of the babies died because my test was incorrect? For the first time in my medical career, I noticed the inherent risk of making necessary decisions with incomplete information.

The rest of medical school and residency cemented my initial observation. I was trapped in a high-risk game of life and death. Suddenly, every small decision I made was infinitely important. Choose correctly and your patient lives; choose incorrectly and they could die.

As time passed, the potential downside of every decision became more and more obvious. In order to not kill my patients, I realized I needed to question, test, and modify my most fundamental beliefs to be more consistent with objective reality. Medicine was more than a profession; it was the art of making decisions without all the facts.

At first, I simply observed like I did with John from the Introduction. After years of focused observation in medical school, I organized my observations into patterns. I wasn't making any decisions yet, but I was still participating (and learning). In residency, my learning accelerated by a factor of a thousand. I validated those patterns by making my own decisions under appropriate supervision. Finally, I engineered strategies to thrive in my new uncertain environment. This book contains those observations, patterns, and strategies.

Additionally, the book serves as an insurance policy against the extinction of anesthesiologists as experts. If the standard of physician-led care is washed away by the shortsighted pursuit of "efficiency," I want to preserve our wisdom for future generations.

I also wanted to share our expertise with those outside of medicine who wish to face uncertainty head-on rather than run from it. I suspect its content is broadly applicable outside the operating room. Black Swans are objective knowledge: they exist whether we think they do or not.

My initial experience in my laboratory made me realize I no longer had the luxury of living in a make-believe world of what-ifs. I took a necessary risk every time I signed an order, administered a drug, or performed a procedure. For me, studying complex systems wasn't a sterile academic pursuit; it was a messy high-stakes poker game of life and death.

The trouble is, in our modern world we can no longer choose not to participate. Because all of us are a part of at least one complex system, we are all playing this same high-stakes poker game whether we like it or not.

In order to not kill my patients, I needed to commit myself 100% to the mastery of my new uncertain environment. First, I learned to simply survive, and then eventually, I learned how to thrive in uncertainty. Now that you know how to observe synergy, Black Swans, and complex systems, the rest is up to you. In our new uncertain world, we need risk takers willing to see reality and then respond accordingly. Our collective future depends on it.

Appendix I

THE UNCERTAINTY CANON

The following books gave me prerequisite knowledge to describe uncertainty in the medical field. Perhaps they might help you recognize, triage, and manage uncertainty in the complex systems of your life.

- Medicine
  - Atul Gawande, MD
    - *Complications: A Surgeon's Notes on an Imperfect Science*
    - *Better: A Surgeon's Notes on Performance*
    - *The Checklist Manifesto: How to Get Things Right*
    - *Being Mortal: Illness, Medicine, and What Matters in the End*
  - H. Gilbert Welch, MD
    - *Overdiagnosed: Making People Sick in the Pursuit of Health*
  - Sandeep Jauhar, MD
    - *Intern: A Doctor's Initiation*
    - *Doctored: The Disillusionment of an American Physician*
    - *Heart: A History*

- Siddhartha Mukherjee, MD
  - *The Emperor of All Maladies: A Biography of Cancer*
  - *The Gene: An Intimate History*
- Victoria Sweet, MD
  - *God's Hotel: A Doctor, a Hospital, and a Pilgrimage to the Heart of Medicine*
- Henry Marsh, MD
  - *Do No Harm: Stories of Life, Death, and Brain Surgery*
- Paul Kalanithi, MD
  - *When Breath Becomes Air*
- Richard Seltzer, MD
  - *Letters to a Young Doctor*
  - *Confessions of a Knife*
- David Rothman
  - *Strangers at the Bedside: A History of How Law and Bioethics Transformed Medical Decision-Making*
- Francis Peabody, MD
  - "The Care of the Patient"
  - *Doctor and Patient*
- Shannon Brownlee
  - *Overtreated: Why Too Much Medicine Is Making Us Sicker and Poorer*
- Rebekah Bernard, MD and Niran Al-Agba, MD
  - *Patients at Risk: The Rise of the Nurse Practitioner and Physician Assistant in Healthcare*
- Social sciences and mathematics (primarily behavioral economics and cognitive psychology)
  - Nassim Taleb
    - *The Black Swan: The Impact of the Highly Improbable*
    - *Antifragile: Things that Gain from Disorder*
    - *Skin in the Game: Hidden Asymmetries in Daily Life*
    - *The Bed of Procrustes: Philosophical and Practical Aphorisms*

- Ray Dalio
  - *Principles: Life and Work*
  - *Principles for Navigating Big Debt Crises*
- Malcolm Gladwell
  - *The Tipping Point: How Little Things Can Make a Big Difference*
  - *Blink: The Power of Thinking without Thinking*
  - *Outliers: The Story of Success*
  - *What the Dog Saw: And Other Adventures*
  - *David and Goliath: Underdogs, Misfits, and the Art of Battling Giants*
  - *Talking to Strangers: What We Should Know about the People We Don't Know*
- Daniel Kahneman
  - *Thinking, Fast and Slow*
- Richard Thaler
  - *Misbehaving: The Making of Behavioral Economics*
  - *Nudge: Improving Decisions about Health, Wealth, and Happiness*
- Gary Klein
  - *Seeing What Others Don't: The Remarkable Ways We Gain Insights*
  - *Sources of Power: How People Make Decisions*
- Al Roth
  - *Who Gets What—and Why: The New Economics of Matchmaking and Market Design*
- Yuval Harari
  - *Sapiens: A Brief History of Humankind*
- David Epstein
  - *Range: Why Generalists Triumph in a Specialized World*
- Jamie Holmes
  - *Nonsense: The Power of Not Knowing*
- Adam Grant

- *Originals: How Non-conformists Move the World*
- Dan Heath
  - *Upstream: The Quest to Solve Problems before They Happen*
- Sun Tzu
  - *The Art of War*
- Alexander Luria
  - *The Mind of a Mnemonist*
- Roger Lowenstein
  - *When Genius Failed: The Rise and Fall of Long-Term Capital Management*
- Steven Levitt and Stephen Dubner
  - *Freakonomics: A Rogue Economist Explains the Hidden Side of Everything*
- Micah Zenko
  - *Red Team: How to Succeed by Thinking like the Enemy*
- Joshua Foer
  - *Moonwalking with Einstein: The Art and Science of Remembering Everything*
- Andrew Newburg, MD
  - *Born to Believe: God, Science, and the Origin of Ordinary and Extraordinary Beliefs*
- Annie Duke
  - *Thinking in Bets: Making Smarter Decisions When You Don't Have All the Facts*

Appendix II

HOW TO BECOME A PHYSICIAN

§ UNDERGRADUATE §

- Completion of an undergraduate degree by the time medical school starts
- Completion of basic science classes
  - General chemistry, biology, organic chemistry, physics, sometimes calculus
  - These classes are not abridged like those taken for health sciences and nursing majors. They are versions taken by those who major in those fields
  - A GPA of 3.7 or more is necessary for admission to most medical schools
  - A poor GPA will hinder your selection
- Medical College Admissions Test (MCAT)
  - Six-hour test of abstraction relating to the medical sciences and humanities
  - A poor MCAT score will hinder your selection
- Applicants must have extensive research, volunteering, entrepreneurial, and extracurricular interests in addition to their academic success

§ MEDICAL SCHOOL §

- Basic science years (two)
  - Written exams in anatomy, histology, physiology, biochemistry, immunology, pathophysiology, and psychiatry
  - Course volume approximately eight to ten undergraduate degrees
  - Almost all medical students complete extensive volunteering, research, and extracurricular involvement in addition to their academic coursework
  - 50 to 100 hours per week
  - Must pass all classes or cannot move on to third year
  - Take USMLE STEP 1 at end. Cannot move on to third year if failed
- Clinical years (two)
  - Third year: Required rotations in internal medicine, pediatrics, family medicine, surgery, neurology, psychiatry, and OB/GYN
    - 50 to 100 hours per week
    - Monthly exams in clerkships
    - Continue longitudinal research, volunteering, and extracurricular activities
    - At end of third year, take USMLE STEP 2 exam
  - Fourth year: Required subinternship, other required rotations, and electives
    - Apply to residency
    - Additional medical school exams per medical school requirements

§ RESIDENCY §

- Intern year (one year)
  - 12 months of rotations in a variety of fields
  - 50 to 100 hours per week
  - Take USMLE STEP 3. Must pass to get a medical license

- Two to six additional years depending on specialty
  - Internal medicine, emergency medicine, pediatrics are three years total
  - Anesthesiology is four years total
  - Neurosurgery is seven years total
  - 50 to 100 hours per week
  - Yearly in-service exam
  - Required research project. Many residents do additional longitudinal research in residency
  - At end, take written board exam
  - Some specialties such as anesthesiology and surgery require additional oral board exams

§ FELLOWSHIP §

- One to three years of optional subspecialty training
- Almost all require research projects
- 50 to 100 hours per week
- Board exam at end

Total time: 11–17 years

Total supervised clinical training hours: 15,000–28,000

Acknowledgments

Writing a book is a team sport. And I have an impressive team behind me.

First and most importantly, I would like to thank my parents.

My mother, Patricia McLeish, instilled positive convexity in me before I knew what it was called. My discipline, intelligence, and kindness are reflections of her. There is no way I can pay you back, but I hope you know I understand.

My stepfather, Jim McLeish, taught me the meaning of the word *dad*. One day, I hope I can guide my own children as you guided me.

In addition to my parents, I had the support of a few other families. The Pitts family: Sandra and Brent, who helped raise me. Cheryl Shearer, who always gave me tough love when I needed it. The Tollon family: Jamie and Tammy who mentored me on and off the soccer field. And of course the Norgaards: Caleb, Stephanie, Elizabeth, Kurt, Sandy, Kreg, and Joel, who accepted me into their family the first day I met them.

§

If I have seen further, it is by standing on the shoulders of Giants. My teachers, professors, and mentors challenged me to grow into the best version of myself. My success is a function of their wisdom and guidance rather than my individual abilities.

First among them, I would like to thank John Biegun, my fifth grade science teacher, who taught me curiosity was an asset rather than a liability.

In high school, Todd Henderson taught me how to study history, Mia Davila instilled discipline, Noelle Collis literally transformed her classroom into a crime scene, and Kurt Ernst proved drawing a perfect circle is indeed possible. Richard Kreinbring taught me how to write by embracing adversity rather than running from it.

My undergraduate chemistry professors Drs. Craig Taylor and Roman Dembinski taught chemistry at the highest level and accepted no excuses. Dr. Art Bull guided me when I was deciding what to do with my life. Dr. Nessan Kerrigan took me under his wing as an undergraduate organic chemistry researcher. My critical thinking skills were honed in his laboratory at night and on weekends. I also had the privilege to work for Sara Webb in the Oakland University Orientation and New Student Programs office. The first day I met her, she told me, "I'm the best boss you will ever have." She was right.

§

In medical school, I was taught by master physicians at the bedside and in the laboratory. The following deserve special mention: Drs. Patrick Hines, Diane Levine, Chetna Jinjuvadia, Ayman

Soubani, Anna Ledgerwood, and Charles Lucas. They taught me physicians are part artisan, part practical scientist, and part diplomat.

My first attendings in residency were surgeons who taught me as one of their own. I owe a debt of gratitude to Drs. Nicholas Nissen, Nicolas Melo, Rodrigo Alban, Rex Chung, Monica Jain, Galinos Bamparas, Daniel Margulies, Matthew Bloom, Eric Ley, Charles Moon, Milton Little, Carol Lin, and Phillip Fleshner. Their work ethic, integrity, and accountability profoundly influenced me as an intern. They transformed an enthusiastic medical student into a real doctor.

My anesthesia co-residents and I spent countless hours together in the operating room, in the ICU, and on call. We saw the best and worst of each other as we grew throughout residency. Without them, I would not be who I am today.

I also had the privilege of rotating with residents from other specialties. My experiences with them gave me the perspective to write this book. I owe a special debt of gratitude to my co-residents in general surgery, internal medicine, neurosurgery, orthopaedic surgery, and critical care for sharing their expertise with me.

During my anesthesiology years, I had teachers and mentors who prioritized my education, including Drs. Laura Zung, Kaveh Navab, Nicola D'Attellis, Manxu Zhao, Stephen Yang, Daniel Sullivan, Robert Wong, Moody Makar, Terrance Lai, Brian Mendelson, Jonathan Hausman, David Sisco, Gabriel Pollock, Avi Gereboff, Vivek Sharma, Anahat Dhillon, Robert Naruse, Taz Yusufali, Omar Durra, Nadeem Hamid, and Alice Vijjeswarapu. They taught me how to assess risk, prevent complications, and make lifesaving decisions during uncertainty.

I documented our countless adventures (and misadventures) in the process of writing this book. I wish I could have included them all, but books have a finite length. The most painful part of the process was choosing which ones to include and which to leave out.

Dr. Roya Yumul, my program director, treated me and my co-residents as her own children. Her high expectations and dedication to our education will benefit us for the rest of our lives; she was our *dura mater*, Latin for "tough mother."

§

In terms of writing, the most important thing I did was seek out high-quality people to criticize my ideas. I quickly learned only 10% of what I wrote was worth keeping. If my writing is high quality it is because I have high-quality editors who recognized the good 10% even when I couldn't see it myself.

Dr. Adam Sawyer introduced me to the philosophy of science and epistemology. Our lively discussions in medical school gave my initial observations the structure they needed to grow into a book.

Before there was a book, there were unorganized rants, poor grammar, and awkward metaphors. Taylor Boykins read all of the initial nonsense and told me what was valuable. Sarah Draugelis and Dr. Jeff Weigers gave me additional insight into the early drafts. Martin Salgo photographed me for the front and back covers. Ariel Weber supported and encouraged me throughout the never-ending writing process.

Publishing books is not cheap. I received financial support from Ariel Weber, Roscoe, Matt Palmer, Andre Latour, AJ Magee, Stephen Lovell, Taylor Boykins, and Chris Lahar. They were willing to put their skin in the game from the beginning.

My publisher, Scribe Media, contributed to the title, designed the cover, facilitated my voice as an author, polished my grammar, and guided me through the business of publishing. Without their expertise, this book would not exist. I would like to thank Jericho Westendorf, Kayla Sokol, Rachael Brandenburg, and John Mannion for their patience as I navigated the publishing process for the first time.

Last, I would like to thank Dr. Pamela Williams for showing me the joy of being a doctor. She was the first person who encouraged me to write about medicine.

About the Author

NABIL OTHMAN, MD, is an anesthesiologist in Los Angeles, California. He earned his bachelor's degree in biochemistry from Oakland University in Rochester, Michigan, followed by his medical degree at Wayne State University in Detroit, Michigan. Currently, he is in his final year of anesthesiology residency at Cedars Sinai Medical Center. After residency, he will complete a critical care fellowship at the Texas Heart Institute. When he is not an indentured servant in the hospital, he enjoys CrossFit, telling everyone he knows about CrossFit, and planning dangerous hikes in Hawaii with his college roommates. He blogs at www.airwaybagelcoffee.com.

9 781544 521060